SYSTEMS & STRUCTURES 2nd Edition

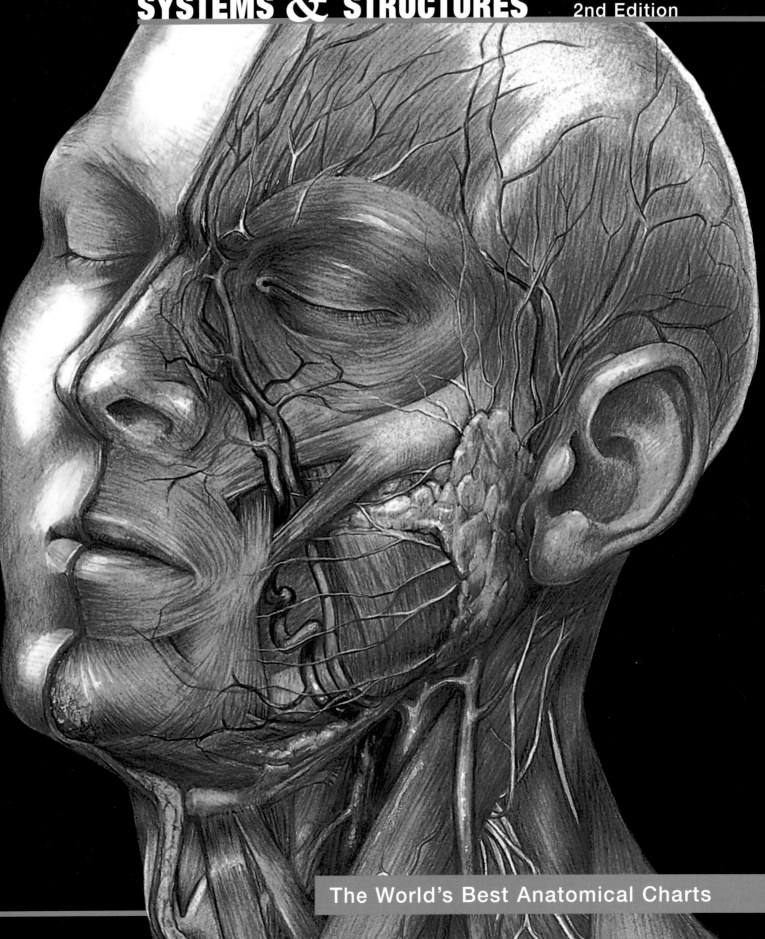

The World's Best Anatomical Charts

CONTENTS

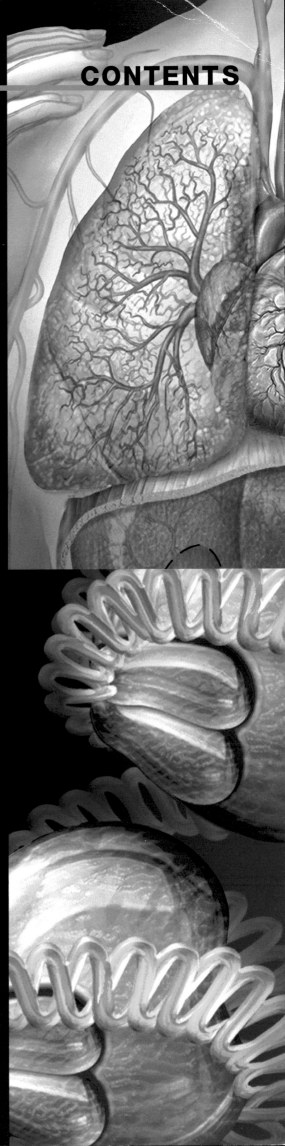

Published by Anatomical Chart Company
A division of Lippincott Williams & Wilkins • A Wolters Kluwer Health Company • Skokie, IL USA

Copyright © 2000, 2005 Lippincott Williams & Wilkins

2nd Edition
ISBN: 1-58779-892-1

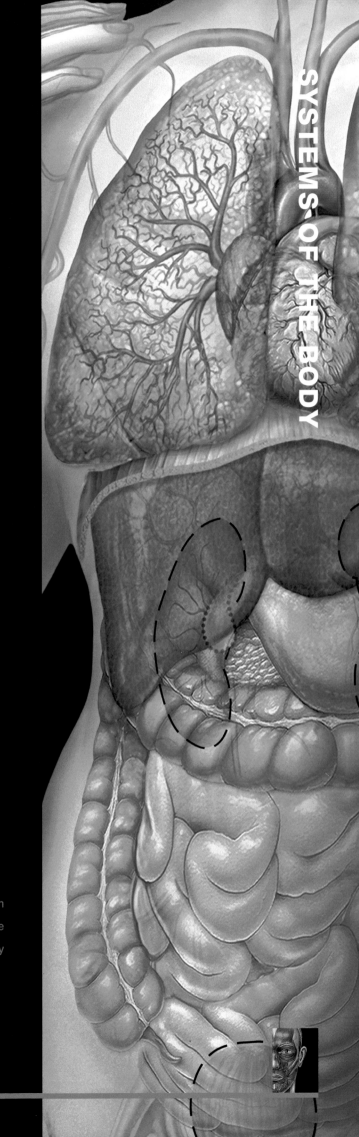

SYSTEMS OF THE BODY

The Digestive System

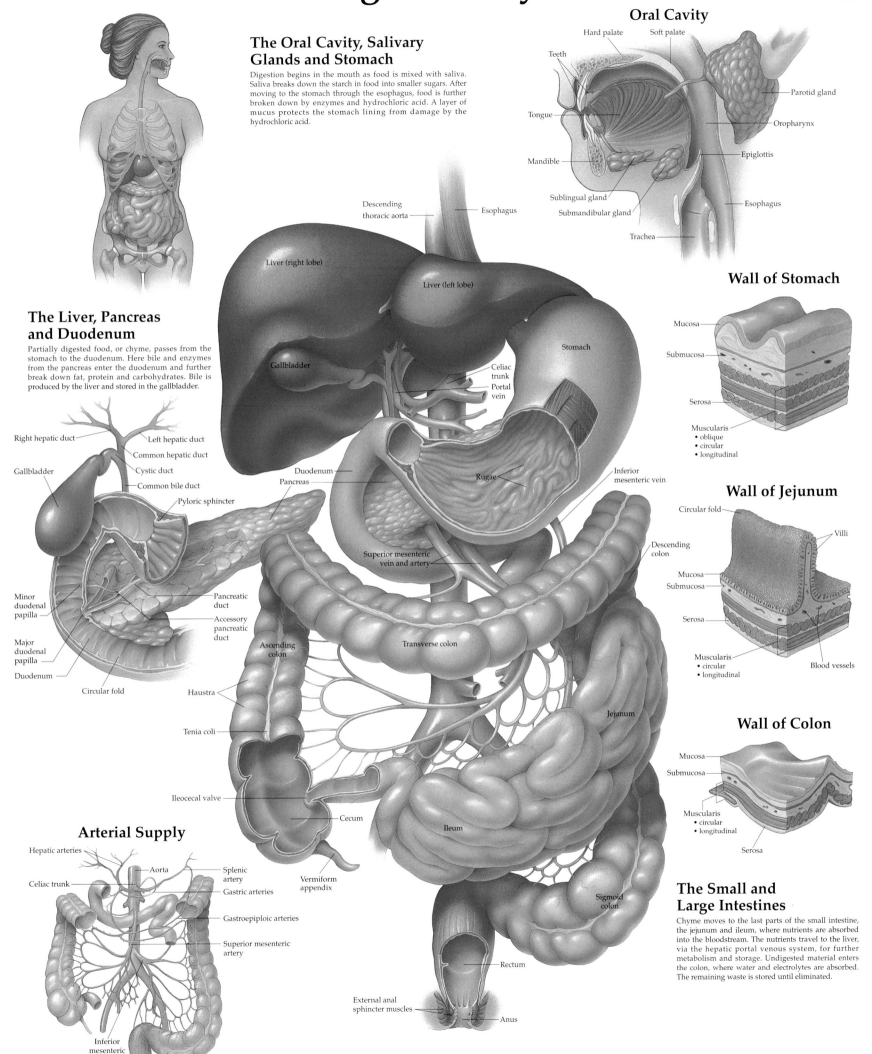

The Oral Cavity, Salivary Glands and Stomach

Digestion begins in the mouth as food is mixed with saliva. Saliva breaks down the starch in food into smaller sugars. After moving to the stomach through the esophagus, food is further broken down by enzymes and hydrochloric acid. A layer of mucus protects the stomach lining from damage by the hydrochloric acid.

Oral Cavity

Hard palate · Soft palate · Teeth · Tongue · Parotid gland · Oropharynx · Mandible · Epiglottis · Sublingual gland · Submandibular gland · Esophagus · Trachea

The Liver, Pancreas and Duodenum

Partially digested food, or chyme, passes from the stomach to the duodenum. Here bile and enzymes from the pancreas enter the duodenum and further break down fat, protein and carbohydrates. Bile is produced by the liver and stored in the gallbladder.

Right hepatic duct · Left hepatic duct · Common hepatic duct · Gallbladder · Cystic duct · Common bile duct · Pyloric sphincter · Minor duodenal papilla · Pancreatic duct · Accessory pancreatic duct · Major duodenal papilla · Duodenum · Circular fold

Descending thoracic aorta · Esophagus · Liver (right lobe) · Liver (left lobe) · Stomach · Gallbladder · Celiac trunk · Portal vein · Duodenum · Pancreas · Rugae · Inferior mesenteric vein · Superior mesenteric vein and artery · Descending colon · Ascending colon · Transverse colon · Haustra · Tenia coli · Jejunum · Ileocecal valve · Cecum · Ileum · Vermiform appendix · Sigmoid colon · Rectum · External anal sphincter muscles · Anus

Wall of Stomach

Mucosa · Submucosa · Serosa · Muscularis
• oblique
• circular
• longitudinal

Wall of Jejunum

Circular fold · Villi · Mucosa · Submucosa · Serosa · Blood vessels · Muscularis
• circular
• longitudinal

Wall of Colon

Mucosa · Submucosa · Muscularis
• circular
• longitudinal
· Serosa

Arterial Supply

Hepatic arteries · Aorta · Splenic artery · Celiac trunk · Gastric arteries · Gastroepiploic arteries · Superior mesenteric artery · Inferior mesenteric artery

The Small and Large Intestines

Chyme moves to the last parts of the small intestine, the jejunum and ileum, where nutrients are absorbed into the bloodstream. The nutrients travel to the liver, via the hepatic portal venous system, for further metabolism and storage. Undigested material enters the colon, where water and electrolytes are absorbed. The remaining waste is stored until eliminated.

The Endocrine System

Thyroid and Parathyroid Glands

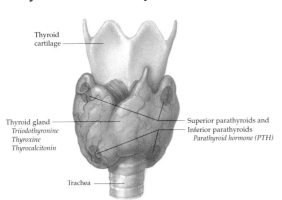

- Thyroid cartilage
- Thyroid gland
  - *Triiodothyronine*
  - *Thyroxine*
  - *Thyrocalcitonin*
- Superior parathyroids and Inferior parathyroids
  - *Parathyroid hormone (PTH)*
- Trachea

Pineal Gland

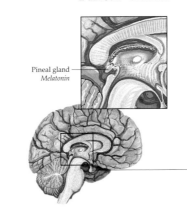

- Pineal gland
  - *Melatonin*

Pituitary Gland and Hypothalamus

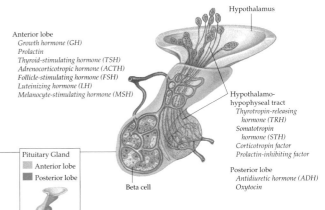

- Hypothalamus
- Anterior lobe
  - *Growth hormone (GH)*
  - *Prolactin*
  - *Thyroid-stimulating hormone (TSH)*
  - *Adrenocorticotropic hormone (ACTH)*
  - *Follicle-stimulating hormone (FSH)*
  - *Luteinizing hormone (LH)*
  - *Melanocyte-stimulating hormone (MSH)*
- Hypothalamo-hypophyseal tract
  - *Thyrotropin-releasing hormone (TRH)*
  - *Somatotropin hormone (STH)*
  - *Corticotropin factor*
  - *Prolactin-inhibiting factor*
- Beta cell
- Posterior lobe
  - *Antidiuretic hormone (ADH)*
  - *Oxytocin*

Pituitary Gland
- Anterior lobe
- Posterior lobe

Thymus Gland

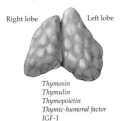

- Right lobe
- Left lobe
- *Thymosin*
- *Thymulin*
- *Thymopoietin*
- *Thymic-humoral factor*
- *IGF-1*

Heart

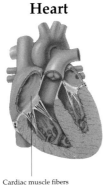

- Cardiac muscle fibers (from the right atrium)
  - *Atrial natriuretic peptide (ANP)*

Stomach, Duodenum, and Jejunum

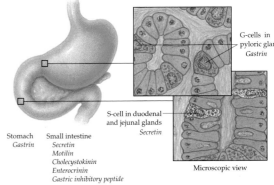

- G-cells in pyloric glands
  - *Gastrin*
- S-cell in duodenal and jejunal glands
  - *Secretin*
- Stomach
  - *Gastrin*
- Small intestine
  - *Secretin*
  - *Motilin*
  - *Cholecystokinin*
  - *Enterocrinin*
  - *Gastric inhibitory peptide*

Microscopic view

Adrenal Glands

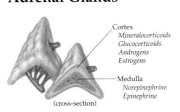

- Cortex
  - *Mineralocorticoids*
  - *Glucocorticoids*
  - *Androgens*
  - *Estrogens*
- Medulla
  - *Norepinephrine*
  - *Epinephrine*

(cross-section)

Pancreas

- Common bile duct
- Pancreatic duct
- Alpha cell
- Beta cell
- Delta cell
- Islet of Langerhans
  - *Glucagon*
  - *Insulin*
  - *Somatostatin*
  - *Pancreatic polypeptide*

Microscopic view

Kidney

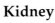

- Kidney
  - *Prostaglandins*
  - *Erythropoietin*
  - *Renin*
- Juxtaglomerular apparatus
- Glomerulus

Microscopic view

Ovary

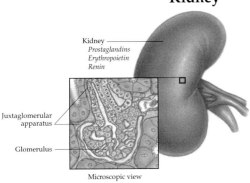

- Fimbria
- Site of ruptured follicle
- Fallopian tube
- Maturing follicles
- Ovary
  - *Estrogen*
  - *Progesterone*
- Follicular fluid
- Corpus luteum
- Developing follicles

(cross-section)

Testes

- Epididymis
- Efferent ducts of epididymis
- Seminiferous tubule
  - *Androgen-binding protein*
  - *A small amount of estrogen*
- Leydig cells
  - *Testosterone*
  - *Androsterone*

(cross-section)

Microscopic view

Placental Hormones
(from uterus during pregnancy)

- *Chorionic gonadotropins*
- *Progesterone*
- *Estrogen*
- *Relaxin*

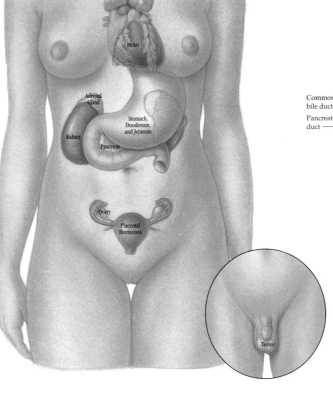

Body figure labels:
- Pineal Gland
- Pituitary Gland
- Thyroid and Parathyroid Glands
- Thymus Gland
- Heart
- Adrenal Gland
- Kidney
- Stomach, Duodenum, and Jejunum
- Pancreas
- Ovary
- Placental Hormones
- Testes

Note: Italicized words represent hormones.

©2005 Anatomical Chart Company Lippincott Williams & Wilkins

The Female Reproductive System

Ovum
(Unfertilized)
100-150μm diameter

- Nucleus
- Nucleolus
- Ooplasm
- Zona pellucida
- Corona radiata
- Polar body

Ovary, Fallopian Tube, Uterus and Vagina

- Fallopian tube
- Isthmus
- Ampulla
- Infundibulum
- Fimbria
- Abdominal opening of fallopian tube
- Secondary oocyte
- Corpus luteum
- Fundus of uterus
- Suspensory ligament of ovary
- Ovarian ligament
- Ovary
- Vesicular appendix
- Cavity of uterus
- Uterus:
  - Perimetrium
  - Myometrium
  - Endometrium
- Broad ligament
- Internal uterine opening
- Cervix
- Cervical canal
- External uterine opening
- Vagina
- Labium minus

The Female Pelvic Organs
(Sagittal section)

L5

- Suspensory ligament of ovary
- Ovary
- Fallopian tube
- Ovarian ligament
- Round ligament
- Median umbilical ligament
- Urinary bladder
- Pubic symphysis
- Urethra
- Clitoris
- Prepuce of clitoris
- Urethral orifice
- Labium minus
- Labium majus
- Vaginal orifice
- Sacrum
- Ureter
- Rectum
- Uterus
- Posterior fornix of vagina
- Rectouterine pouch
- Cervix
- Levator ani muscle
- Vagina
- Anus

The Female Perineum

- Pubic symphysis
- Prepuce
- Urethral orifice
- Ischiocavernous muscle
- Bulbospongiosus muscle
- Vaginal orifice
- Deep transverse perineal muscle
- Ischial tuberosity
- Levator ani muscle
- Anus
- External anal sphincter
- Gluteus maximus muscle
- Clitoris:
  - Body
  - Glans
  - Crus
- Labium majus
- Labium minus
- Pudendal nerve

Ovary

- Primary oocyte
- Developing follicles
- Mature graafian follicle
- Antrum filled with liquor folliculi
- Expulsion of secondary oocyte
- Corpus luteum

Uterus

Ovulation

- Endometrium:
  - Stratum functionale
  - Stratum basale
- Myometrium
- Uterine gland
- Venous lacunae
- Endometrial vein
- Spiral artery
- Basal artery
- Arcuate artery

Day 0	4	14	26	28
Menstrual phase	Proliferative phase	Secretory phase	Premenstrual phase	

The Menstrual Cycle

The menstrual cycle occurs during the reproductive period from puberty through menopause in response to rhythmic variations of hormones. The endometrial lining of the uterus proliferates in preparation for implantation of a fertilized egg. In the absence of pregnancy the lining is shed with some bleeding through the vagina.

Menopause

Menopause, the gradual interruption and cessation of menstrual cycles, occurs at about 45 to 50 years of age. It is associated with the depletion of oocytes in the ovary and subsequent decline of estrogen levels.

The Lymphatic System

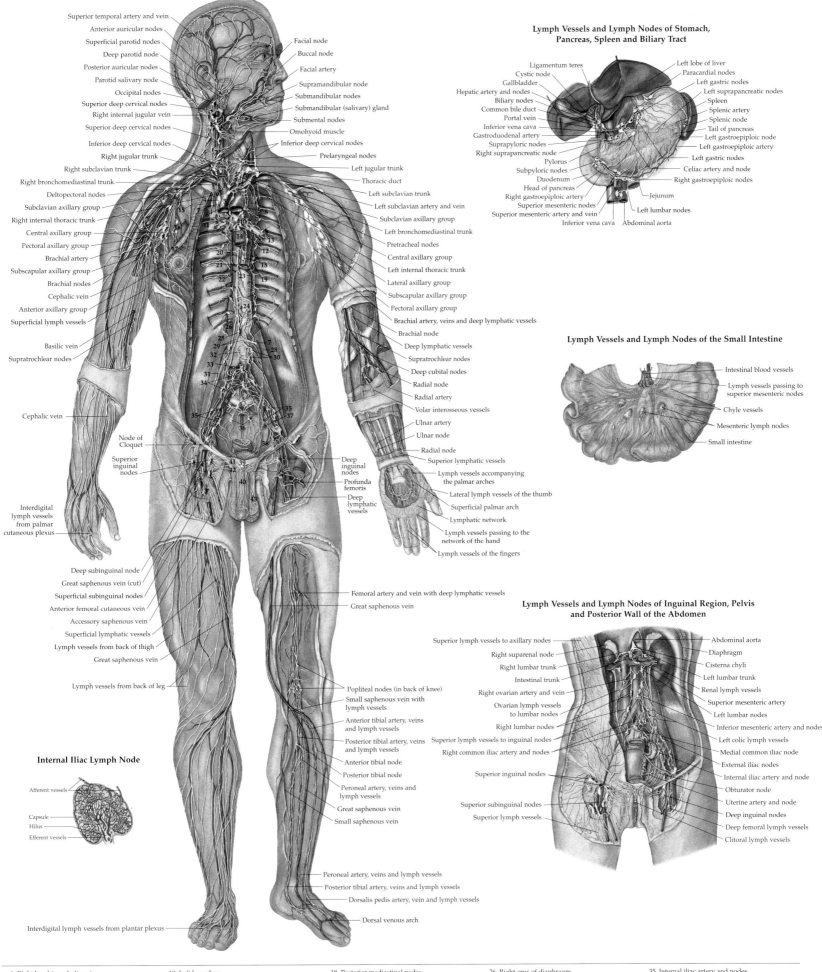

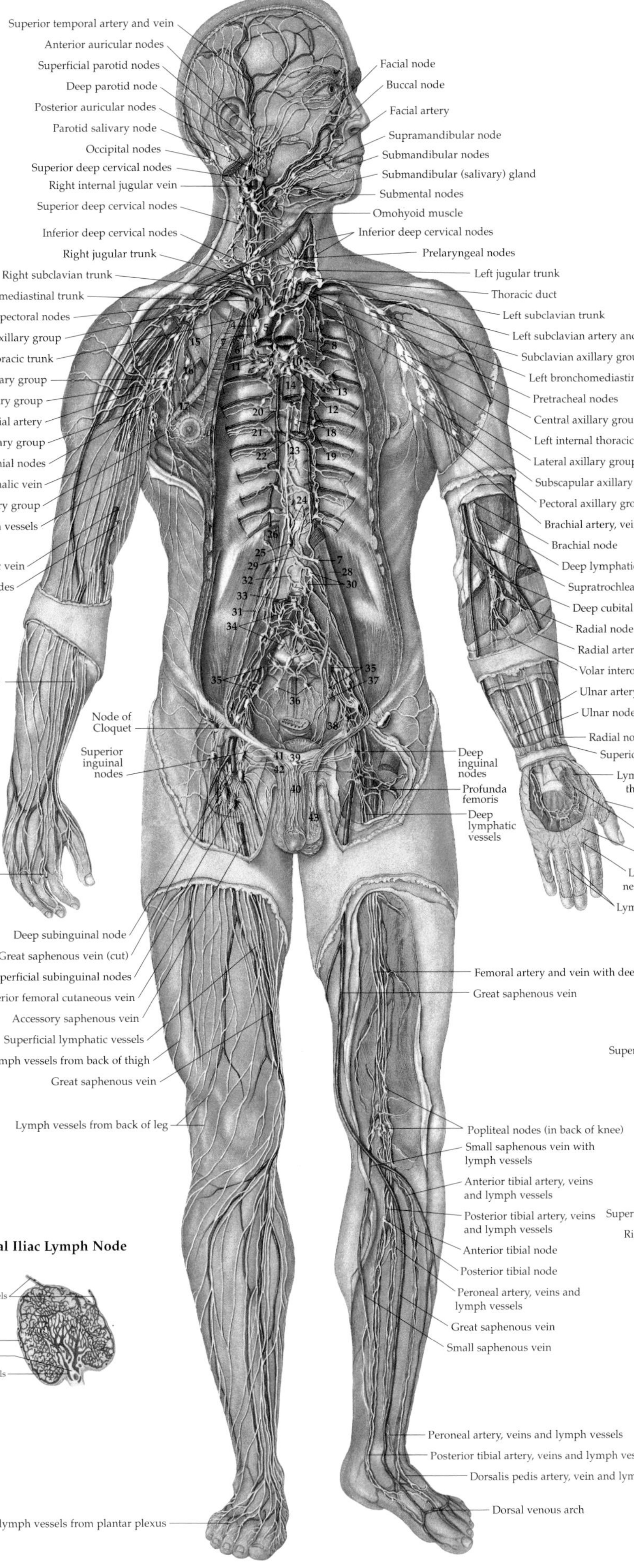
Superior temporal artery and vein
Anterior auricular nodes
Superficial parotid nodes
Deep parotid node
Posterior auricular nodes
Parotid salivary node
Occipital nodes
Superior deep cervical nodes
Right internal jugular vein
Superior deep cervical nodes
Inferior deep cervical nodes
Right jugular trunk
Right subclavian trunk
Right bronchomediastinal trunk
Deltopectoral nodes
Subclavian axillary group
Right internal thoracic trunk
Central axillary group
Pectoral axillary group
Brachial artery
Subscapular axillary group
Brachial nodes
Cephalic vein
Anterior axillary group
Superficial lymph vessels
Basilic vein
Supratrochlear nodes
Cephalic vein
Node of Cloquet
Superior inguinal nodes
Interdigital lymph vessels from palmar cutaneous plexus
Deep subinguinal node
Great saphenous vein (cut)
Superficial subinguinal nodes
Anterior femoral cutaneous vein
Accessory saphenous vein
Superficial lymphatic vessels
Lymph vessels from back of thigh
Great saphenous vein
Lymph vessels from back of leg
Interdigital lymph vessels from plantar plexus
Facial node
Buccal node
Facial artery
Supramandibular node
Submandibular nodes
Submandibular (salivary) gland
Submental nodes
Omohyoid muscle
Inferior deep cervical nodes
Prelaryngeal nodes
Left jugular trunk
Thoracic duct
Left subclavian trunk
Left subclavian artery and vein
Subclavian axillary group
Left bronchomediastinal trunk
Pretracheal nodes
Central axillary group
Left internal thoracic trunk
Lateral axillary group
Subscapular axillary group
Pectoral axillary group
Brachial artery, veins and deep lymphatic vessels
Brachial node
Deep lymphatic vessels
Supratrochlear nodes
Deep cubital nodes
Radial node
Radial artery
Volar interosseous vessels
Ulnar artery
Ulnar node
Radial node
Superior lymphatic vessels
Lymph vessels accompanying the palmar arches
Lateral lymph vessels of the thumb
Superficial palmar arch
Lymphatic network
Lymph vessels passing to the network of the hand
Lymph vessels of the fingers
Deep inguinal nodes
Profunda femoris
Deep lymphatic vessels
Femoral artery and vein with deep lymphatic vessels
Great saphenous vein
Popliteal nodes (in back of knee)
Small saphenous vein with lymph vessels
Anterior tibial artery, veins and lymph vessels
Posterior tibial artery, veins and lymph vessels
Anterior tibial node
Posterior tibial node
Peroneal artery, veins and lymph vessels
Great saphenous vein
Small saphenous vein
Peroneal artery, veins and lymph vessels
Posterior tibial artery, veins and lymph vessels
Dorsalis pedis artery, vein and lymph vessels
Dorsal venous arch

Lymph Vessels and Lymph Nodes of Stomach, Pancreas, Spleen and Biliary Tract

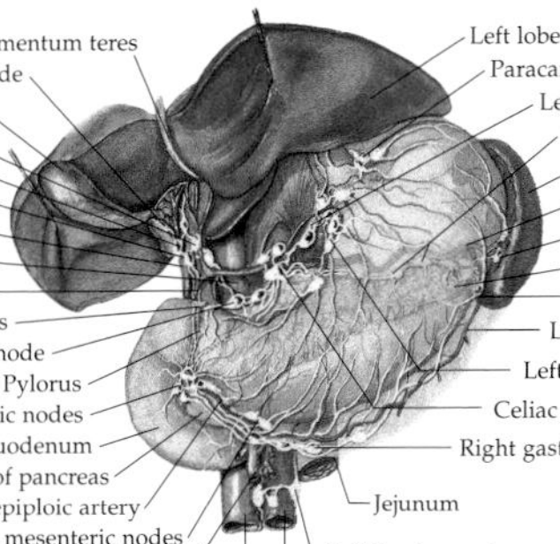
Ligamentum teres
Cystic node
Gallbladder
Hepatic artery and nodes
Biliary nodes
Common bile duct
Portal vein
Inferior vena cava
Gastroduodenal artery
Suprapyloric nodes
Right suprapancreatic node
Pylorus
Subpyloric nodes
Duodenum
Head of pancreas
Right gastroepiploic artery
Superior mesenteric nodes
Superior mesenteric artery and vein
Inferior vena cava
Abdominal aorta
Left lumbar nodes
Jejunum
Left lobe of liver
Paracardial nodes
Left gastric nodes
Left suprapancreatic nodes
Spleen
Splenic artery
Splenic node
Tail of pancreas
Left gastroepiploic node
Left gastroepiploic artery
Left gastric nodes
Celiac artery and node
Right gastroepiploic nodes

Lymph Vessels and Lymph Nodes of the Small Intestine

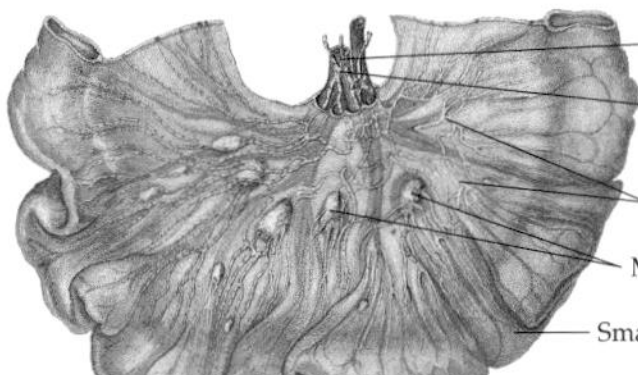
Intestinal blood vessels
Lymph vessels passing to superior mesenteric nodes
Chyle vessels
Mesenteric lymph nodes
Small intestine

Lymph Vessels and Lymph Nodes of Inguinal Region, Pelvis and Posterior Wall of the Abdomen

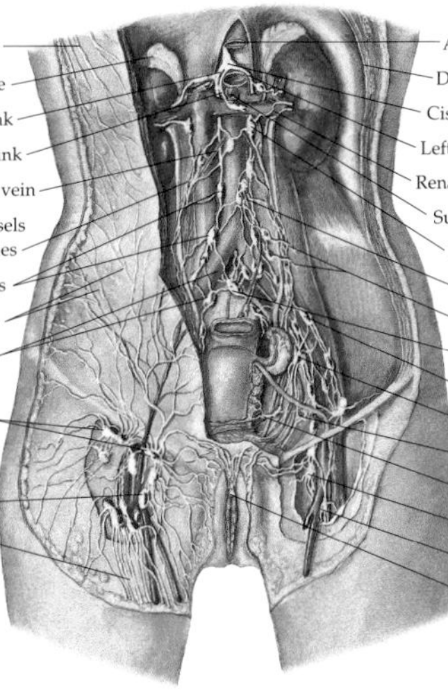
Superior lymph vessels to axillary nodes
Right suparenal node
Right lumbar trunk
Intestinal trunk
Right ovarian artery and vein
Ovarian lymph vessels to lumbar nodes
Right lumbar nodes
Superior lymph vessels to inguinal nodes
Right common iliac artery and nodes
Superior inguinal nodes
Superior subinguinal nodes
Superior lymph vessels
Abdominal aorta
Diaphragm
Cisterna chyli
Left lumbar trunk
Renal lymph vessels
Superior mesenteric artery
Left lumbar nodes
Inferior mesenteric artery and nodes
Left colic lymph vessels
Medial common iliac node
External iliac nodes
Internal iliac artery and node
Obturator node
Uterine artery and node
Deep inguinal nodes
Deep femoral lymph vessels
Clitoral lymph vessels

Internal Iliac Lymph Node

Afferent vessels
Capsule
Hilus
Efferent vessels

1. Right brachiocephalic vein
2. Left brachiocephalic vein
3. Left common carotid artery
4. Anterior superior mediastinal nodes
5. Superior vena cava
6. Right cardiac lymph branch
7. Internal thoracic node
8. Node of ligamentum arteriosum
9. Right bronchus
10. Left bronchus
11. Right tracheobronchial nodes
12. Left tracheobronchial nodes
13. Right and left bronchopulmonary nodes
14. Esophagus
15. Internal thoracic lymph vessel ending in subclavicular nodes
16. Interpectoral nodes
17. Lymph vessels from deep part of breast
18. Posterior mediastinal nodes
19. Intercostal nodes and lymph vessels
20. Azygos vein
21. Thoracic duct
22. Thoracic aorta
23. Hemiazygos vein
24. Descending right and left intercostal lymph trunks
25. Cisterna chyli
26. Right crus of diaphragm
27. Intestinal trunk
28. Psoas major muscle
29. Right and left lumbar trunks
30. Lumbar nodes
31. Testicular lymph vessels
32. Retroaortic node (lumbar nodes)
33. Preaortic node (lumbar nodes)
34. Common iliac nodes
35. Internal iliac artery and nodes
36. Sacral nodes
37. Lymph vessels to internal iliac nodes
38. Obturator vessels and nerve
39. Presymphysial node
40. Collecting lymph vessels from glans penis
41. Superior lymph vessels from the penis
42. Lymph vessels from the scrotum
43. Lymph vessels of testis and epididymus

The Male Reproductive System

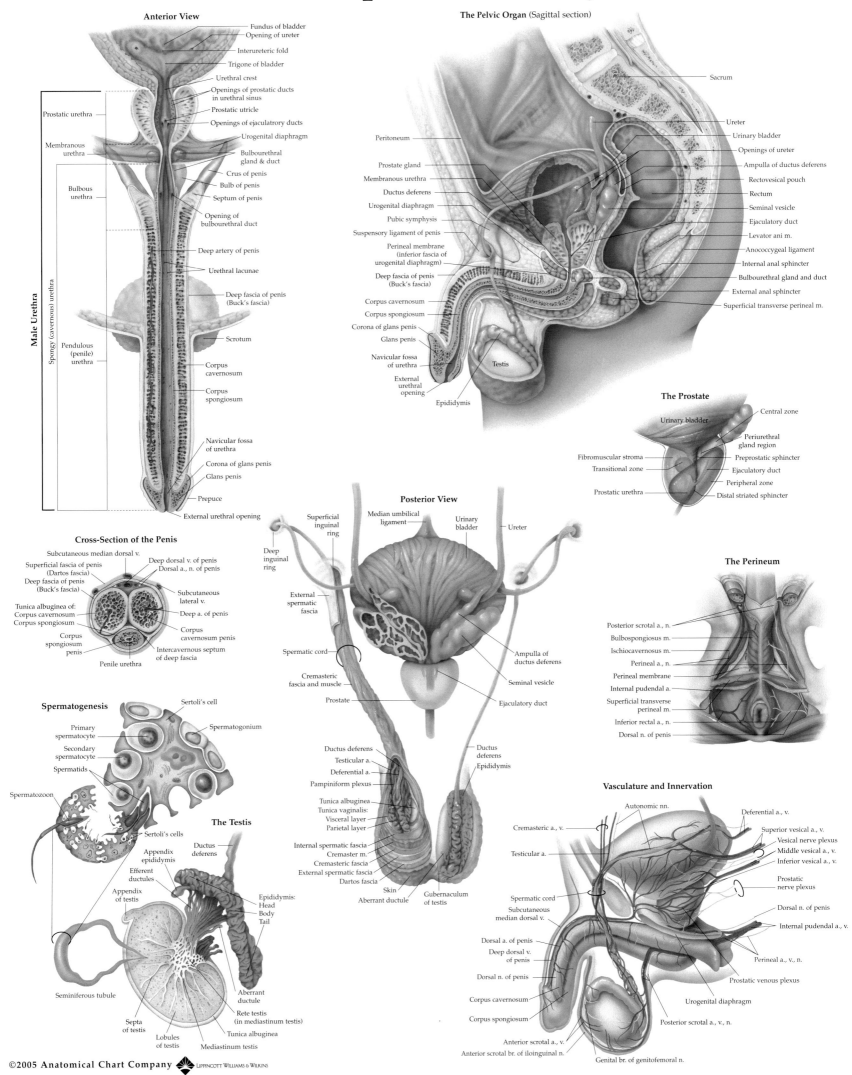

Anterior View

Fundus of bladder
Opening of ureter
Interureteric fold
Trigone of bladder
Urethral crest
Openings of prostatic ducts in urethral sinus
Prostatic utricle
Openings of ejaculatory ducts
Urogenital diaphragm
Bulbourethral gland & duct
Crus of penis
Bulb of penis
Septum of penis
Opening of bulbourethral duct
Deep artery of penis
Urethral lacunae
Deep fascia of penis (Buck's fascia)
Scrotum
Corpus cavernosum
Corpus spongiosum
Navicular fossa of urethra
Corona of glans penis
Glans penis
Prepuce
External urethral opening

Prostatic urethra
Membranous urethra
Bulbous urethra
Pendulous (penile) urethra
Spongy (cavernous) urethra
Male Urethra

The Pelvic Organ (Sagittal section)

Sacrum
Ureter
Urinary bladder
Openings of ureter
Ampulla of ductus deferens
Rectovesical pouch
Rectum
Seminal vesicle
Ejaculatory duct
Levator ani m.
Anococcygeal ligament
Internal anal sphincter
Bulbourethral gland and duct
External anal sphincter
Superficial transverse perineal m.

Peritoneum
Prostate gland
Membranous urethra
Ductus deferens
Urogenital diaphragm
Pubic symphysis
Suspensory ligament of penis
Perineal membrane (inferior fascia of urogenital diaphragm)
Deep fascia of penis (Buck's fascia)
Corpus cavernosum
Corpus spongiosum
Corona of glans penis
Glans penis
Navicular fossa of urethra
External urethral opening
Epididymis
Testis

The Prostate

Central zone
Periurethral gland region
Preprostatic sphincter
Ejaculatory duct
Peripheral zone
Distal striated sphincter
Urinary bladder
Fibromuscular stroma
Transitional zone
Prostatic urethra

Cross-Section of the Penis

Subcutaneous median dorsal v.
Superficial fascia of penis (Dartos fascia)
Deep fascia of penis (Buck's fascia)
Tunica albuginea of: Corpus cavernosum, Corpus spongiosum
Corpus spongiosum penis
Penile urethra
Dorsal a., n. of penis
Deep dorsal v. of penis
Subcutaneous lateral v.
Deep a. of penis
Corpus cavernosum penis
Intercavernous septum of deep fascia

Posterior View

Superficial inguinal ring
Median umbilical ligament
Urinary bladder
Ureter
Deep inguinal ring
External spermatic fascia
Spermatic cord
Cremasteric fascia and muscle
Prostate
Ampulla of ductus deferens
Seminal vesicle
Ejaculatory duct

The Perineum

Posterior scrotal a., n.
Bulbospongiosus m.
Ischiocavernosus m.
Perineal a., n.
Perineal membrane
Internal pudendal a.
Superficial transverse perineal m.
Inferior rectal a., n.
Dorsal n. of penis

Spermatogenesis

Sertoli's cell
Primary spermatocyte
Secondary spermatocyte
Spermatids
Spermatogonium
Spermatozoon
Sertoli's cells

The Testis

Ductus deferens
Appendix epididymis
Appendix of testis
Efferent ductules
Epididymis: Head, Body, Tail
Seminiferous tubule
Aberrant ductule
Septa of testis
Lobules of testis
Mediastinum testis
Rete testis (in mediastinum testis)
Tunica albuginea

Ductus deferens
Testicular a.
Deferential a.
Pampiniform plexus
Tunica albuginea
Tunica vaginalis: Visceral layer, Parietal layer
Internal spermatic fascia
Cremaster m.
Cremasteric fascia
External spermatic fascia
Dartos fascia
Skin
Aberrant ductule
Ductus deferens
Epididymis
Gubernaculum of testis

Vasculature and Innervation

Autonomic nn.
Cremasteric a., v.
Testicular a.
Spermatic cord
Subcutaneous median dorsal v.
Dorsal a. of penis
Deep dorsal v. of penis
Dorsal n. of penis
Corpus cavernosum
Corpus spongiosum
Anterior scrotal a., v.
Anterior scrotal br. of ilioinguinal n.
Genital br. of genitofemoral n.
Posterior scrotal a., v., n.
Urogenital diaphragm
Prostatic venous plexus
Perineal a., v., n.
Internal pudendal a., v.
Dorsal n. of penis
Prostatic nerve plexus
Inferior vesical a., v.
Middle vesical a., v.
Vesical nerve plexus
Superior vesical a., v.
Deferential a., v.

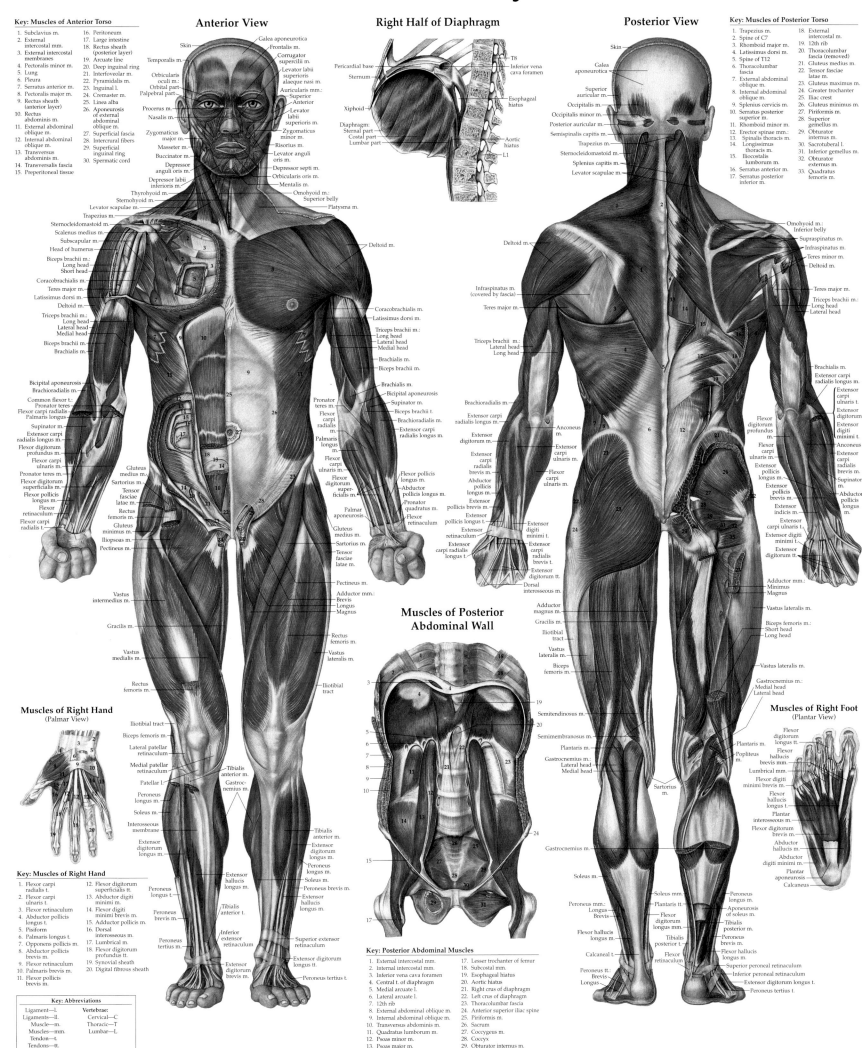

Anterior View

Right Half of Diaphragm

Posterior View

Muscles of Posterior Abdominal Wall

Muscles of Right Hand
(Palmar View)

Muscles of Right Foot
(Plantar View)

Key: Muscles of Anterior Torso

1. Subclavius m.
2. External intercostal mm.
3. External intercostal membranes
4. Pectoralis minor m.
5. Lung
6. Pleura
7. Serratus anterior m.
8. Pectoralis major m.
9. Rectus sheath (anterior layer)
10. Rectus abdominis m.
11. External abdominal oblique m.
12. Internal abdominal oblique m.
13. Transversus abdominis m.
14. Transversalis fascia
15. Preperitoneal tissue
16. Peritoneum
17. Large intestine
18. Rectus sheath (posterior layer)
19. Arcuate line
20. Deep inguinal ring
21. Interfoveolar m.
22. Pyramidalis m.
23. Inguinal l.
24. Cremaster m.
25. Linea alba
26. Aponeurosis of external abdominal oblique m.
27. Superficial fascia
28. Intercrural fibers
29. Superficial inguinal ring
30. Spermatic cord

Key: Muscles of Posterior Torso

1. Trapezius m.
2. Spine of C7
3. Rhomboid major m.
4. Latissimus dorsi m.
5. Spine of T12
6. Thoracolumbar fascia
7. External abdominal oblique m.
8. Internal abdominal oblique m.
9. Splenius cervicis m.
10. Serratus posterior superior m.
11. Rhomboid minor m.
12. Erector spinae mm.:
13. Spinalis thoracis m.
14. Longissimus thoracis m.
15. Iliocostalis lumborum m.
16. Serratus anterior m.
17. Serratus posterior inferior m.
18. External intercostal m.
19. 12th rib
20. Thoracolumbar fascia (removed)
21. Gluteus medius m.
22. Tensor fasciae latae m.
23. Gluteus maximus m.
24. Greater trochanter
25. Iliac crest
26. Gluteus minimus m.
27. Piriformis m.
28. Superior gemellus m.
29. Obturator internus m.
30. Sacrotuberal l.
31. Inferior gemellus m.
32. Obturator externus m.
33. Quadratus femoris m.

Key: Muscles of Right Hand

1. Flexor carpi radialis t.
2. Flexor carpi ulnaris t.
3. Flexor retinaculum
4. Abductor pollicis longus t.
5. Pisiform
6. Palmaris longus t.
7. Opponens pollicis m.
8. Abductor pollicis brevis m.
9. Flexor retinaculum
10. Palmaris brevis m.
11. Flexor pollicis brevis m.
12. Flexor digitorum superficialis tt.
13. Abductor digiti minimi m.
14. Flexor digiti minimi brevis m.
15. Adductor pollicis m.
16. Dorsal interosseous m.
17. Lumbrical m.
18. Flexor digitorum profundus tt.
19. Synovial sheath
20. Digital fibrous sheath

Key: Posterior Abdominal Muscles

1. External intercostal mm.
2. Internal intercostal mm.
3. Inferior vena cava foramen
4. Central t. of diaphragm
5. Medial arcuate l.
6. Lateral arcuate l.
7. 12th rib
8. External abdominal oblique m.
9. Internal abdominal oblique m.
10. Transversus abdominis m.
11. Quadratus lumborum m.
12. Psoas minor m.
13. Psoas major m.
14. Iliacus m.
15. Inguinal l.
16. Iliopsoas m.
17. Lesser trochanter of femur
18. Subcostal mm.
19. Esophageal hiatus
20. Aortic hiatus
21. Right crus of diaphragm
22. Left crus of diaphragm
23. Thoracolumbar fascia
24. Anterior superior iliac spine
25. Piriformis m.
26. Sacrum
27. Coccygeus m.
28. Coccyx
29. Obturator internus m.
30. Levator ani m.
31. Obturator externus m.

Key: Abbreviations

Ligament—l.
Ligaments—ll.
Muscle—m.
Muscles—mm.
Tendon—t.
Tendons—tt.

Vertebrae:
Cervical—C
Thoracic—T
Lumbar—L

The Female Muscular System

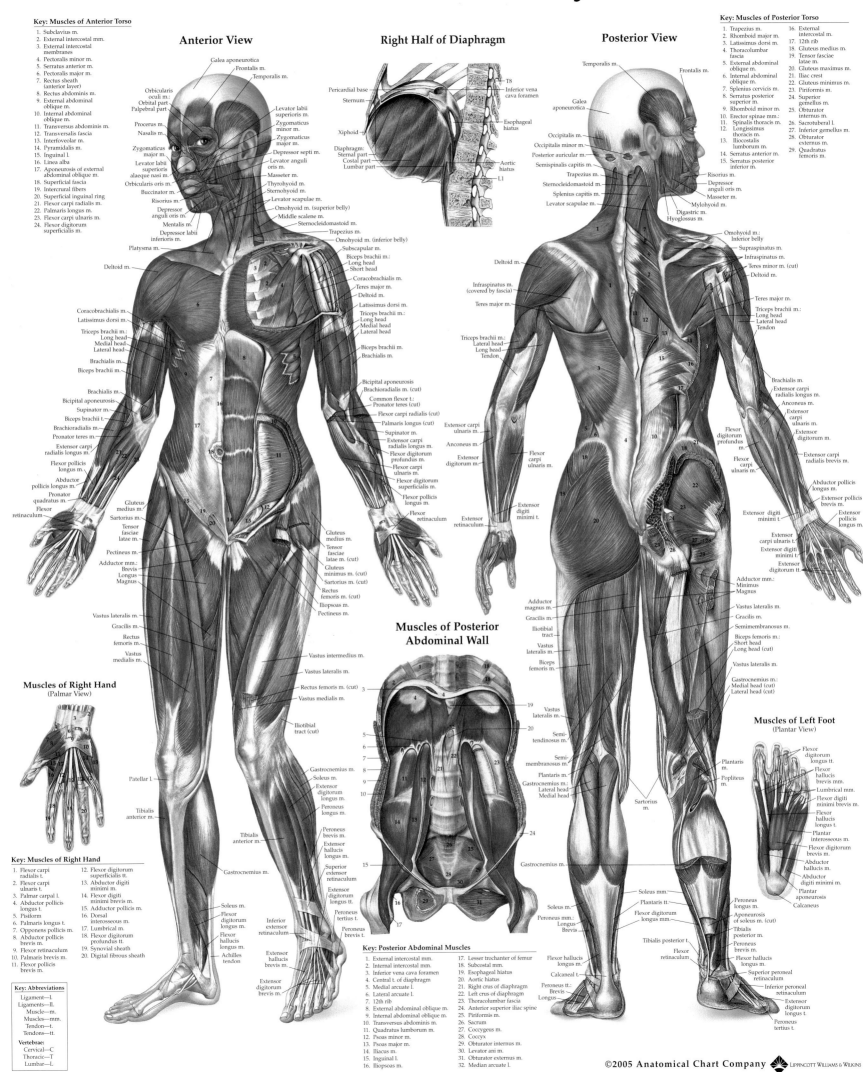

Key: Muscles of Anterior Torso
1. Subclavius m.
2. External intercostal mm.
3. External intercostal membranes
4. Pectoralis minor m.
5. Serratus anterior m.
6. Pectoralis major m.
7. Rectus sheath (anterior layer)
8. Rectus abdominis m.
9. External abdominal oblique m.
10. Internal abdominal oblique m.
11. Transversus abdominis m.
12. Transversalis fascia
13. Interfoveolar m.
14. Pyramidalis m.
15. Inguinal l.
16. Linea alba
17. Aponeurosis of external abdominal oblique m.
18. Superficial fascia
19. Intercrural fibers
20. Superficial inguinal ring
21. Flexor carpi radialis m.
22. Palmaris longus m.
23. Flexor carpi ulnaris m.
24. Flexor digitorum superficialis m.

Anterior View

Right Half of Diaphragm

Posterior View

Key: Muscles of Posterior Torso
1. Trapezius m.
2. Rhomboid major m.
3. Latissimus dorsi m.
4. Thoracolumbar fascia
5. External abdominal oblique m.
6. Internal abdominal oblique m.
7. Splenius cervicis m.
8. Serratus posterior superior m.
9. Rhomboid minor m.
10. Erector spinae mm.
11. Spinalis thoracis m.
12. Longissimus thoracis m.
13. Iliocostalis lumborum m.
14. Serratus anterior m.
15. Serratus posterior inferior m.
16. External intercostal m.
17. 12th rib
18. Gluteus medius m.
19. Tensor fasciae latae m.
20. Gluteus maximus m.
21. Iliac crest
22. Gluteus minimus m.
23. Piriformis m.
24. Superior gemellus m.
25. Obturator internus m.
26. Sacrotuberal l.
27. Inferior gemellus m.
28. Obturator externus m.
29. Quadratus femoris m.

Anterior View labels
Galea aponeurotica
Frontalis m.
Temporalis m.
Orbicularis oculi m.
Orbital part
Palpebral part
Levator labii superioris m.
Zygomaticus minor m.
Zygomaticus major m.
Procerus m.
Nasalis m.
Depressor septi m.
Zygomaticus major m.
Levator anguli oris m.
Levator labii superioris alaeque nasi m.
Masseter m.
Orbicularis oris m.
Thyrohyoid m.
Buccinator m.
Sternohyoid m.
Risorius m.
Levator scapulae m.
Depressor anguli oris m.
Omohyoid m. (superior belly)
Mentalis m.
Middle scalene m.
Depressor labii inferioris m.
Sternocleidomastoid m.
Platysma m.
Trapezius m.
Omohyoid m. (inferior belly)
Deltoid m.
Biceps brachii m.:
Long head
Short head
Coracobrachialis m.
Teres major m.
Deltoid m.
Latissimus dorsi m.
Triceps brachii m.:
Long head
Medial head
Lateral head
Biceps brachii m.
Brachialis m.
Coracobrachialis m.
Latissimus dorsi m.
Triceps brachii m.:
Long head
Medial head
Lateral head
Brachialis m.
Biceps brachii m.
Bicipital aponeurosis
Brachioradialis m. (cut)
Common flexor t.:
Pronator teres (cut)
Brachialis m.
Bicipital aponeurosis
Supinator m.
Biceps brachii t.
Flexor carpi radialis (cut)
Palmaris longus (cut)
Brachioradialis m.
Pronator teres m.
Supinator m.
Extensor carpi radialis longus m.
Extensor carpi radialis longus m.
Flexor digitorum profundus m.
Flexor carpi ulnaris m.
Flexor digitorum superficialis m.
Flexor pollicis longus m.
Flexor retinaculum
Flexor pollicis longus m.
Abductor pollicis longus m.
Pronator quadratus m.
Flexor retinaculum
Gluteus medius m.
Tensor fasciae latae m.
Sartorius m.
Tensor fasciae latae m. (cut)
Gluteus minimus m. (cut)
Sartorius m. (cut)
Rectus femoris m. (cut)
Iliopsoas m.
Pectineus m.
Pectineus m.
Adductor mm.:
Brevis
Longus
Magnus
Vastus lateralis m.
Gracilis m.
Rectus femoris m.
Vastus medialis m.
Vastus intermedius m.
Vastus lateralis m.
Rectus femoris m. (cut)
Vastus medialis m.
Iliotibial tract (cut)
Patellar l.
Gastrocnemius m.
Soleus m.
Extensor digitorum longus m.
Peroneus longus m.
Tibialis anterior m.
Peroneus brevis m.
Extensor hallucis longus m.
Tibialis anterior m.
Superior extensor retinaculum
Extensor digitorum longus m.
Gastrocnemius m.
Peroneus tertius t.
Inferior extensor retinaculum
Soleus m.
Flexor digitorum longus m.
Flexor hallucis longus m.
Peroneus brevis m.
Achilles tendon
Extensor hallucis brevis m.
Extensor digitorum brevis m.

Right Half of Diaphragm labels
Pericardial base
Sternum
Xiphoid
Diaphragm:
Sternal part
Costal part
Lumbar part
T8
Inferior vena cava foramen
Esophageal hiatus
Aortic hiatus
L1

Posterior View labels
Temporalis m.
Frontalis m.
Occipitalis m.
Galea aponeurotica
Occipitalis minor m.
Posterior auricular m.
Semispinalis capitis m.
Trapezius m.
Risorius m.
Depressor anguli oris m.
Masseter m.
Mylohyoid m.
Digastric m.
Hyoglossus m.
Sternocleidomastoid m.
Splenius capitis m.
Levator scapulae m.
Omohyoid m.:
Inferior belly
Supraspinatus m.
Infraspinatus m.
Teres minor m. (cut)
Deltoid m.
Deltoid m.
Infraspinatus m. (covered by fascia)
Teres major m.
Teres major m.
Triceps brachii m.:
Long head
Lateral head
Tendon
Triceps brachii m.:
Lateral head
Long head
Tendon
Brachialis m.
Extensor carpi radialis longus m.
Anconeus m.
Extensor carpi ulnaris m.
Extensor digitorum m.
Extensor carpi ulnaris m.
Anconeus m.
Extensor digitorum m.
Flexor carpi ulnaris m.
Flexor digitorum profundus m.
Extensor carpi radialis brevis m.
Flexor carpi ulnaris m.
Extensor digiti minimi t.
Extensor retinaculum
Abductor pollicis longus m.
Extensor pollicis brevis m.
Extensor digiti minimi t.
Extensor pollicis longus m.
Extensor carpi ulnaris t.
Extensor digiti minimi t.
Extensor digitorum tt.
Adductor mm.:
Minimus
Magnus
Vastus lateralis m.
Gracilis m.
Semimembranosus m.
Biceps femoris m.:
Short head
Long head (cut)
Vastus lateralis m.
Gastrocnemius m.:
Medial head (cut)
Lateral head (cut)
Adductor magnus m.
Gracilis m.
Iliotibial tract
Vastus lateralis m.
Biceps femoris m.
Semitendinosus m.
Semimembranosus m.
Plantaris m.
Gastrocnemius m.:
Lateral head
Medial head
Sartorius m.
Plantaris m.
Popliteus m.
Gastrocnemius m.
Soleus m.
Plantaris mm.
Soleus mm.:
Peroneus mm.:
Longus
Brevis
Flexor digitorum longus mm.
Tibialis posterior m.
Flexor retinaculum

Muscles of Posterior Abdominal Wall

Key: Posterior Abdominal Muscles
1. External intercostal mm.
2. Internal intercostal mm.
3. Inferior vena cava foramen
4. Central t. of diaphragm
5. Medial arcuate l.
6. Lateral arcuate l.
7. 12th rib
8. External abdominal oblique m.
9. Internal abdominal oblique m.
10. Transversus abdominis m.
11. Quadratus lumborum m.
12. Psoas minor m.
13. Psoas major m.
14. Iliacus m.
15. Inguinal l.
16. Iliopsoas m.
17. Lesser trochanter of femur
18. Subcostal m.
19. Esophageal hiatus
20. Aortic hiatus
21. Right crus of diaphragm
22. Left crus of diaphragm
23. Thoracolumbar fascia
24. Anterior superior iliac spine
25. Piriformis m.
26. Sacrum
27. Coccygeus m.
28. Coccyx
29. Obturator internus m.
30. Levator ani m.
31. Obturator externus m.
32. Median arcuate l.

Muscles of Right Hand
(Palmar View)

Key: Muscles of Right Hand
1. Flexor carpi radialis t.
2. Flexor carpi ulnaris t.
3. Palmar carpal l.
4. Abductor pollicis longus t.
5. Pisiform
6. Palmaris longus t.
7. Opponens pollicis m.
8. Abductor pollicis brevis m.
9. Flexor retinaculum
10. Palmaris brevis m.
11. Flexor pollicis brevis m.
12. Flexor digitorum superficialis tt.
13. Abductor digiti minimi m.
14. Flexor digiti minimi brevis m.
15. Adductor pollicis m.
16. Dorsal interosseous m.
17. Lumbrical m.
18. Flexor digitorum profundus tt.
19. Synovial sheath
20. Digital fibrous sheath

Muscles of Left Foot
(Plantar View)

Left Foot labels
Flexor digitorum longus tt.
Flexor hallucis brevis mm.
Lumbrical mm.
Flexor digiti minimi brevis m.
Flexor hallucis longus t.
Plantar interosseous m.
Flexor digitorum brevis m.
Abductor hallucis m.
Abductor digiti minimi m.
Plantar aponeurosis
Calcaneus
Peroneus longus m.
Aponeurosis of soleus m. (cut)
Tibialis posterior m.
Peroneus brevis m.
Flexor hallucis longus m.
Superior peroneal retinaculum
Inferior peroneal retinaculum
Extensor digitorum longus t.
Peroneus tertius t.

Key: Abbreviations
Ligament—l.
Ligaments—ll.
Muscle—m.
Muscles—mm.
Tendon—t.
Tendons—tt.

Vertebrae:
Cervical—C
Thoracic—T
Lumbar—L

The Autonomic Nervous System

KEY

1. Lacrimal gland
2. Ciliary ganglion
3. Trigeminal ganglion
4. Otic ganglion
5. Pterygopalatine ganglion
6. Internal carotid plexus
7. Parotid gland
8. Superior cervical ganglion
9. External carotid plexus
10. Submandibular ganglion
11. Carotid body

12. Middle cervical ganglion
13. Inferior cervical ganglion
14. Vagus nerve
15. Aortic lymphatic plexus
16. Cardiopulmonary plexus
17. Deep and superficial cardiac plexus
18. Bronchial branch of vagus nerve
19. Pulmonary plexus
20. Greater splanchnic nerve

21. Esophageal plexus
22. Lesser splanchnic nerve
23. Gastric plexuses
24. Celiac ganglia and plexus
25. Nerve to adrenal gland (medulla)
26. Superior mesenteric ganglion
27. Renal plexus
28. Superior mesenteric plexus
29. Inferior mesenteric ganglion
30. Inferior mesenteric plexus

31. Sacral plexus
32. Pelvic splanchnic nerve
33. Superior hypogastric plexus
34. Inferior hypogastric plexus
35. Vesical plexus
36. Ductus deferens plexus
37. Ganglion impar
38. Pudendal nerve (somatic)
39. Prostatic plexus
40. Dorsal nerve of penis
41. Testicular plexus

Midbrain
Pons
Medulla
Spinal nerves
III
VII
IX
X

Ciliary ganglion
Pterygopalatine ganglion
Submandibular ganglion
Lacrimal gland
Submandibular gland
Sublingual gland
Parotid gland
Otic ganglion

Spinal nerves: C1, C2, C3, C4 — To neck
C5, C6, C7, C8 — To upper limb
T1, T2, T3, T4, T5, T6, T7, T8, T9, T10, T11, T12, L1, L2 — To body wall
L3, L4, L5, S1, S2, S3, S4, S5 — To lower limb
S2, S3, S4, S5 — To perineum

Spinal cord segments: C1–C8, T1–T12, L1–L5, S1–S5, Co1

Superior cervical ganglion
Middle cervical ganglion
Inferior cervical ganglion

Vagus nerve
Larynx
Trachea
Pulmonary nerves
Bronchus
Lung
Cervical cardiac nn.: Superior, Middle, Inferior
Thoracic cardiac nerves
Heart

Celiac ganglia
Greater splanchnic nerve
Lesser and least splanchnic nerve
Aortico-renal ganglia
Superior mesenteric ganglion
Lumbar splanchnic nerves
Inferior mesenteric ganglion
Sympathetic ganglion
Pelvic splanchnic nerve

Liver
Gallbladder
Bile duct
Spleen
Pancreas
Adrenal gland cortex
Kidney
Esophagus
Stomach
Bladder
Prostate
Rectum
Urethra
Uterus
Testis

Colon:
A – Ascending
B – Transverse
C – Descending

KEY

Blue lines - Parasympathetic
Red lines - Sympathetic
Solid lines - Preganglionic motor neuron
Dashed lines - Postganglionic motor neuron
III - Oculomotor nerve
VII - Facial nerve
IX - Glossopharyngeal nerve
X - Vagus nerve

The Nervous System

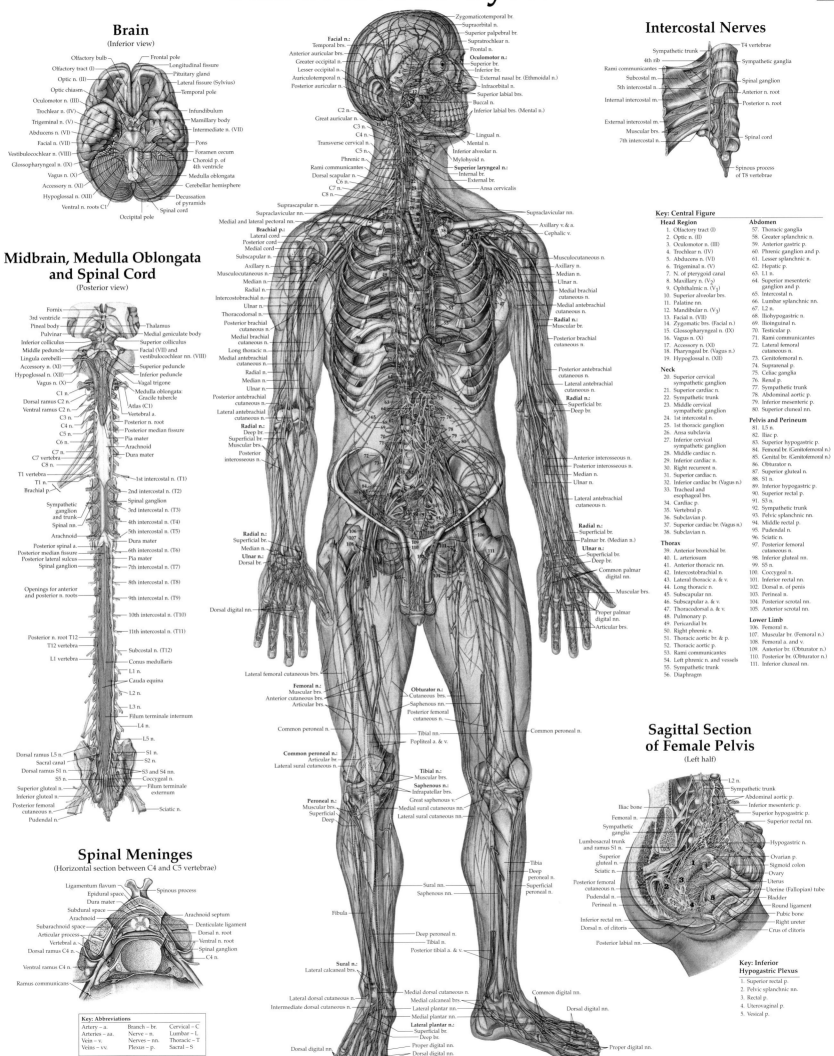

The Respiratory System

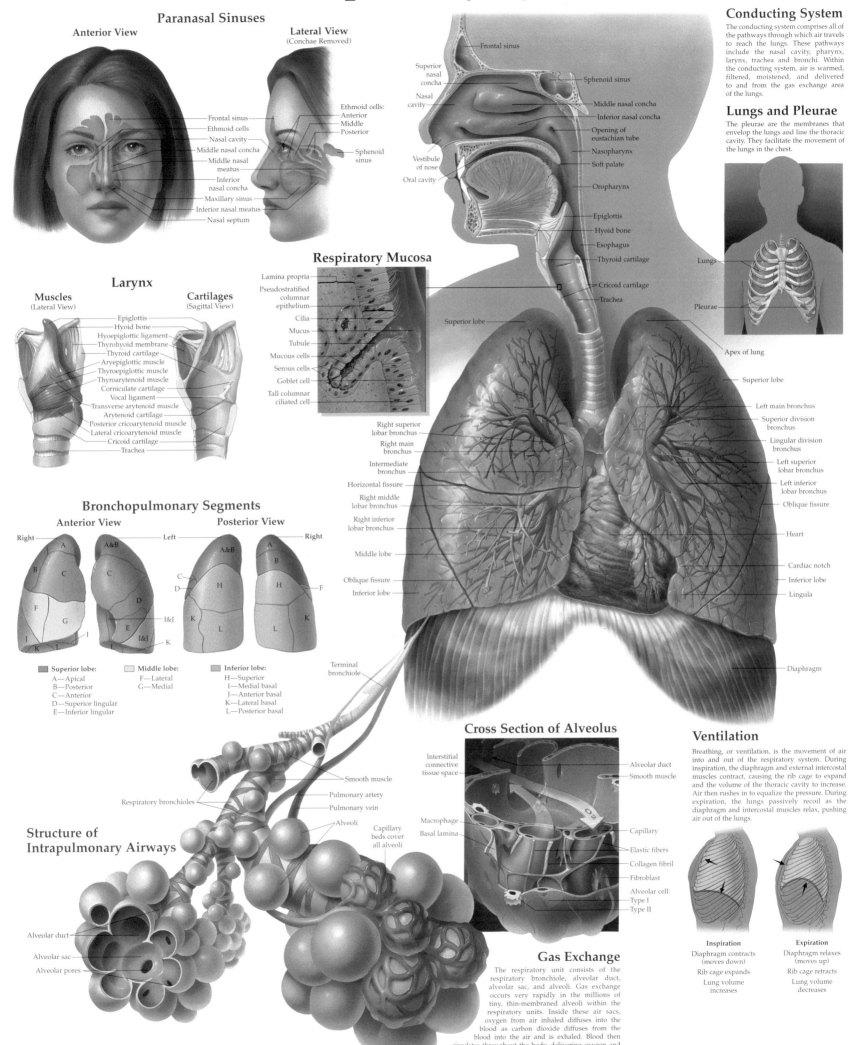

Paranasal Sinuses

Anterior View

- Frontal sinus
- Ethmoid cells
- Nasal cavity
- Middle nasal concha
- Middle nasal meatus
- Inferior nasal concha
- Maxillary sinus
- Inferior nasal meatus
- Nasal septum

Lateral View
(Conchae Removed)

Ethmoid cells:
- Anterior
- Middle
- Posterior
- Sphenoid sinus

Larynx

Muscles
(Lateral View)

Cartilages
(Sagittal View)

- Epiglottis
- Hyoid bone
- Hyoepiglottic ligament
- Thyrohyoid membrane
- Thyroid cartilage
- Aryepiglottic muscle
- Thyroepiglottic muscle
- Thyroarytenoid muscle
- Corniculate cartilage
- Vocal ligament
- Transverse arytenoid muscle
- Arytenoid cartilage
- Posterior cricoarytenoid muscle
- Lateral cricoarytenoid muscle
- Cricoid cartilage
- Trachea

Respiratory Mucosa

- Lamina propria
- Pseudostratified columnar epithelium
- Cilia
- Mucus
- Tubule
- Mucous cells
- Serous cells
- Goblet cell
- Tall columnar ciliated cell

(Central sagittal head/neck section labels)

- Frontal sinus
- Superior nasal concha
- Nasal cavity
- Sphenoid sinus
- Middle nasal concha
- Inferior nasal concha
- Opening of eustachian tube
- Vestibule of nose
- Nasopharynx
- Soft palate
- Oral cavity
- Oropharynx
- Epiglottis
- Hyoid bone
- Esophagus
- Thyroid cartilage
- Cricoid cartilage
- Trachea
- Superior lobe

Conducting System

The conducting system comprises all of the pathways through which air travels to reach the lungs. These pathways include the nasal cavity, pharynx, larynx, trachea and bronchi. Within the conducting system, air is warmed, filtered, moistened, and delivered to and from the gas exchange area of the lungs.

Lungs and Pleurae

The pleurae are the membranes that envelop the lungs and line the thoracic cavity. They facilitate the movement of the lungs in the chest.

- Lungs
- Pleurae
- Apex of lung
- Superior lobe
- Left main bronchus
- Superior division bronchus
- Lingular division bronchus
- Left superior lobar bronchus
- Left inferior lobar bronchus
- Oblique fissure
- Heart
- Cardiac notch
- Inferior lobe
- Lingula
- Diaphragm

- Right superior lobar bronchus
- Right main bronchus
- Intermediate bronchus
- Horizontal fissure
- Right middle lobar bronchus
- Right inferior lobar bronchus
- Middle lobe
- Oblique fissure
- Inferior lobe

Bronchopulmonary Segments

Anterior View

Right — Left

Posterior View

Left — Right

Superior lobe:
- A—Apical
- B—Posterior
- C—Anterior
- D—Superior lingular
- E—Inferior lingular

Middle lobe:
- F—Lateral
- G—Medial

Inferior lobe:
- H—Superior
- I—Medial basal
- J—Anterior basal
- K—Lateral basal
- L—Posterior basal

Structure of Intrapulmonary Airways

- Terminal bronchiole
- Smooth muscle
- Pulmonary artery
- Pulmonary vein
- Respiratory bronchioles
- Alveoli
- Capillary beds cover all alveoli
- Alveolar duct
- Alveolar sac
- Alveolar pores

Cross Section of Alveolus

- Interstitial connective tissue space
- Alveolar duct
- Smooth muscle
- Macrophage
- Basal lamina
- Capillary
- Elastic fibers
- Collagen fibril
- Fibroblast
- Alveolar cell:
  - Type I
  - Type II

Gas Exchange

The respiratory unit consists of the respiratory bronchiole, alveolar duct, alveolar sac, and alveoli. Gas exchange occurs very rapidly in the millions of tiny, thin-membraned alveoli within the respiratory units. Inside these air sacs, oxygen from air inhaled diffuses into the blood as carbon dioxide diffuses from the blood into the air and is exhaled. Blood then circulates throughout the body, delivering oxygen and picking up carbon dioxide, until returning to the lungs to be oxygenated again.

Ventilation

Breathing, or ventilation, is the movement of air into and out of the respiratory system. During inspiration, the diaphragm and external intercostal muscles contract, causing the rib cage to expand and the volume of the thoracic cavity to increase. Air then rushes in to equalize the pressure. During expiration, the lungs passively recoil as the diaphragm and intercostal muscles relax, pushing air out of the lungs.

Inspiration
- Diaphragm contracts (moves down)
- Rib cage expands
- Lung volume increases

Expiration
- Diaphragm relaxes (moves up)
- Rib cage retracts
- Lung volume decreases

The Skeletal System

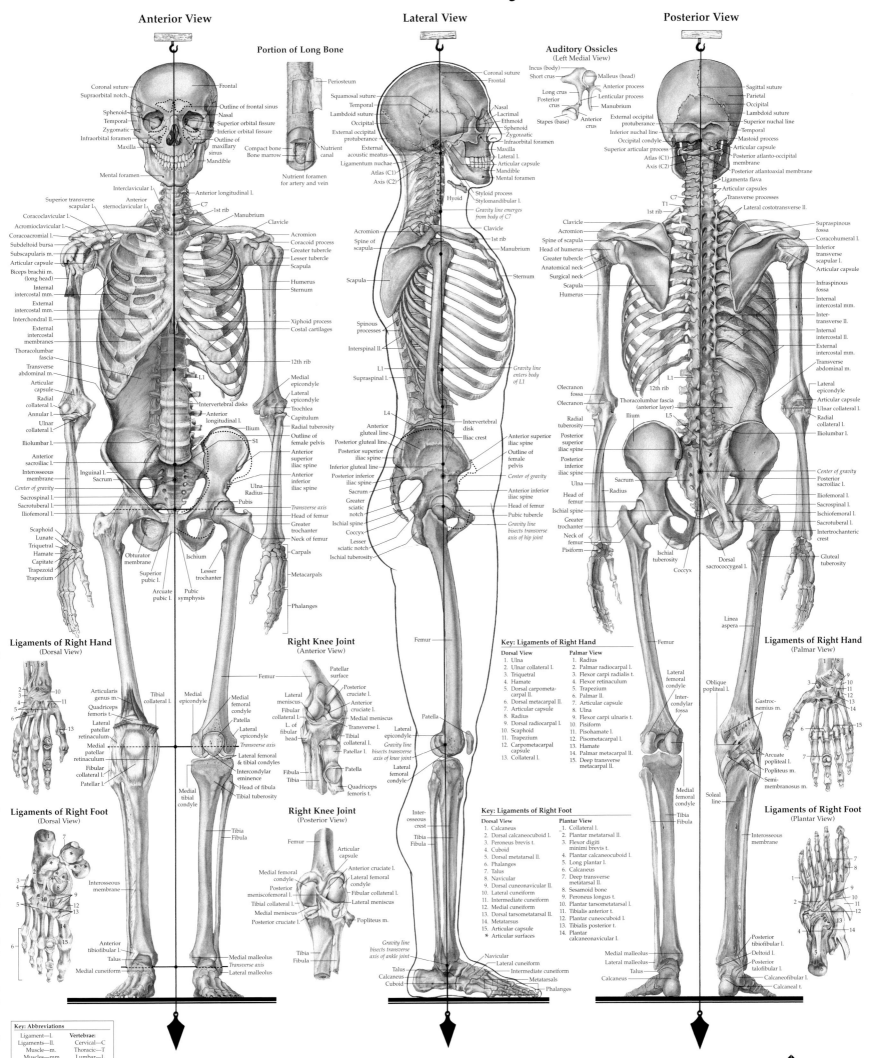

Anterior View

Lateral View

Posterior View

Portion of Long Bone

Auditory Ossicles
(Left Medial View)

Ligaments of Right Hand
(Dorsal View)

Right Knee Joint
(Anterior View)

Key: Ligaments of Right Hand

Dorsal View	Palmar View
1. Ulna	1. Radius
2. Ulnar collateral l.	2. Palmar radiocarpal l.
3. Triquetral	3. Flexor carpi radialis t.
4. Hamate	4. Flexor retinaculum
5. Dorsal carpometa-carpal ll.	5. Trapezium
6. Dorsal metacarpal ll.	6. Palmar ll.
7. Articular capsule	7. Articular capsule
8. Radius	8. Ulna
9. Dorsal radiocarpal l.	9. Flexor carpi ulnaris t.
10. Scaphoid	10. Pisiform
11. Trapezium	11. Pisohamate l.
12. Carpometacarpal capsule	12. Pisometacarpal l.
13. Collateral l.	13. Hamate
	14. Palmar metacarpal ll.
	15. Deep transverse metacarpal l.

Ligaments of Right Hand
(Palmar View)

Ligaments of Right Foot
(Dorsal View)

Right Knee Joint
(Posterior View)

Key: Ligaments of Right Foot

Dorsal View	Plantar View
1. Calcaneus	1. Collateral l.
2. Dorsal calcaneocuboid l.	2. Plantar metatarsal ll.
3. Peroneus brevis t.	3. Flexor digiti minimi brevis t.
4. Cuboid	4. Plantar calcaneocuboid l.
5. Dorsal metatarsal ll.	5. Long plantar l.
6. Phalanges	6. Calcaneus
7. Talus	7. Deep transverse metatarsal ll.
8. Navicular	8. Sesamoid bone
9. Dorsal cuneonavicular ll.	9. Peroneus longus t.
10. Lateral cuneiform	10. Plantar tarsometatarsal l.
11. Intermediate cuneiform	11. Tibialis anterior t.
12. Medial cuneiform	12. Plantar cuneocuboid l.
13. Dorsal tarsometatarsal ll.	13. Tibialis posterior t.
14. Metatarsus	14. Plantar calcaneonavicular l.
15. Articular capsule	
* Articular surfaces	

Ligaments of Right Foot
(Plantar View)

The Urinary Tract

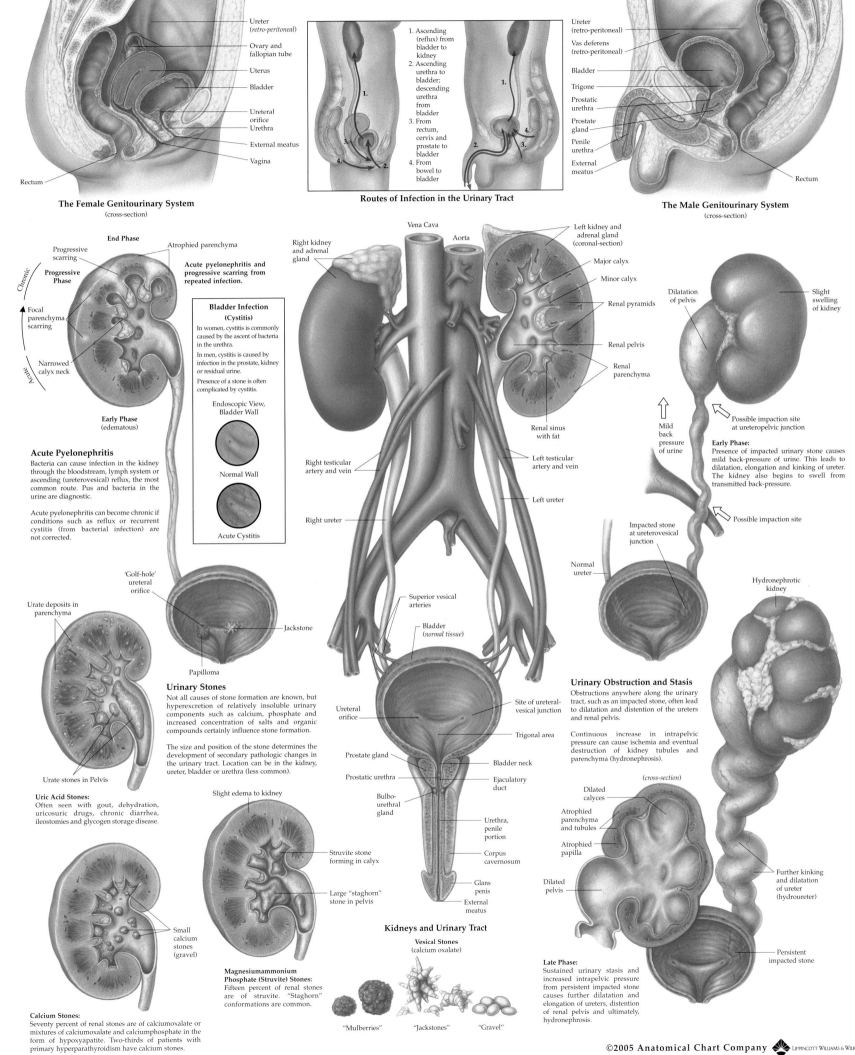

The Female Genitourinary System
(cross-section)

- Ureter (retro-peritoneal)
- Ovary and fallopian tube
- Uterus
- Bladder
- Ureteral orifice
- Urethra
- External meatus
- Vagina
- Rectum

Routes of Infection in the Urinary Tract

1. Ascending (reflux) from bladder to kidney
2. Ascending urethra to bladder; descending urethra from bladder
3. From rectum, cervix and prostate to bladder
4. From bowel to bladder

The Male Genitourinary System
(cross-section)

- Ureter (retro-peritoneal)
- Vas deferens (retro-peritoneal)
- Bladder
- Trigone
- Prostatic urethra
- Prostate gland
- Penile urethra
- External meatus
- Rectum

Acute Pyelonephritis

End Phase
- Progressive scarring
- Atrophied parenchyma

Progressive Phase
Acute pyelonephritis and progressive scarring from repeated infection.

- Focal parenchyma scarring
- Narrowed calyx neck

Early Phase (edematous)

Bacteria can cause infection in the kidney through the bloodstream, lymph system or ascending (ureterovesical) reflux, the most common route. Pus and bacteria in the urine are diagnostic.

Acute pyelonephritis can become chronic if conditions such as reflux or recurrent cystitis (from bacterial infection) are not corrected.

Bladder Infection (Cystitis)

In women, cystitis is commonly caused by the ascent of bacteria in the urethra.

In men, cystitis is caused by infection in the prostate, kidney or residual urine.

Presence of a stone is often complicated by cystitis.

Endoscopic View, Bladder Wall
- Normal Wall
- Acute Cystitis

Urinary Stones

- Urate deposits in parenchyma
- 'Golf-hole' ureteral orifice
- Jackstone
- Papilloma
- Urate stones in Pelvis

Not all causes of stone formation are known, but hyperexcretion of relatively insoluble urinary components such as calcium, phosphate and increased concentration of salts and organic compounds certainly influence stone formation.

The size and position of the stone determines the development of secondary pathologic changes in the urinary tract. Location can be in the kidney, ureter, bladder or urethra (less common).

Uric Acid Stones:
Often seen with gout, dehydration, uricosuric drugs, chronic diarrhea, ileostomies and glycogen storage disease.

Kidneys and Urinary Tract

- Vena Cava
- Aorta
- Right kidney and adrenal gland
- Left kidney and adrenal gland (coronal-section)
- Major calyx
- Minor calyx
- Renal pyramids
- Renal pelvis
- Renal parenchyma
- Renal sinus with fat
- Right testicular artery and vein
- Left testicular artery and vein
- Left ureter
- Right ureter
- Superior vesical arteries
- Bladder (normal tissue)
- Ureteral orifice
- Site of ureteral-vesical junction
- Trigonal area
- Prostate gland
- Bladder neck
- Prostatic urethra
- Ejaculatory duct
- Bulbo-urethral gland
- Urethra, penile portion
- Corpus cavernosum
- Glans penis
- External meatus

Vesical Stones (calcium oxalate)

- "Mulberries"
- "Jackstones"
- "Gravel"

Calcium Stones:
Seventy percent of renal stones are of calciumoxalate or mixtures of calciumoxalate and calciumphosphate in the form of hypoxyapatite. Two-thirds of patients with primary hyperparathyroidism have calcium stones.

- Slight edema to kidney
- Struvite stone forming in calyx
- Large "staghorn" stone in pelvis
- Small calcium stones (gravel)

Magnesiumammonium Phosphate (Struvite) Stones:
Fifteen percent of renal stones are of struvite. "Staghorn" conformations are common.

Urinary Obstruction and Stasis

- Dilatation of pelvis
- Slight swelling of kidney
- Mild back pressure of urine
- Possible impaction site at ureteropelvic junction

Early Phase:
Presence of impacted urinary stone causes mild back-pressure of urine. This leads to dilatation, elongation and kinking of ureter. The kidney also begins to swell from transmitted back-pressure.

- Possible impaction site
- Impacted stone at ureterovesical junction
- Normal ureter

Obstructions anywhere along the urinary tract, such as an impacted stone, often lead to dilatation and distension of the ureters and renal pelvis.

Continuous increase in intrapelvic pressure can cause ischemia and eventual destruction of kidney tubules and parenchyma (hydronephrosis).

- Hydronephrotic kidney
- Dilated calyces
- Atrophied parenchyma and tubules
- Atrophied papilla
- Dilated pelvis
- Further kinking and dilatation of ureter (hydroureter)
- Persistent impacted stone

(cross-section)

Late Phase:
Sustained urinary stasis and increased intrapelvic pressure from persistent impacted stone causes further dilatation and elongation of ureters, distension of renal pelvis and ultimately, hydronephrosis.

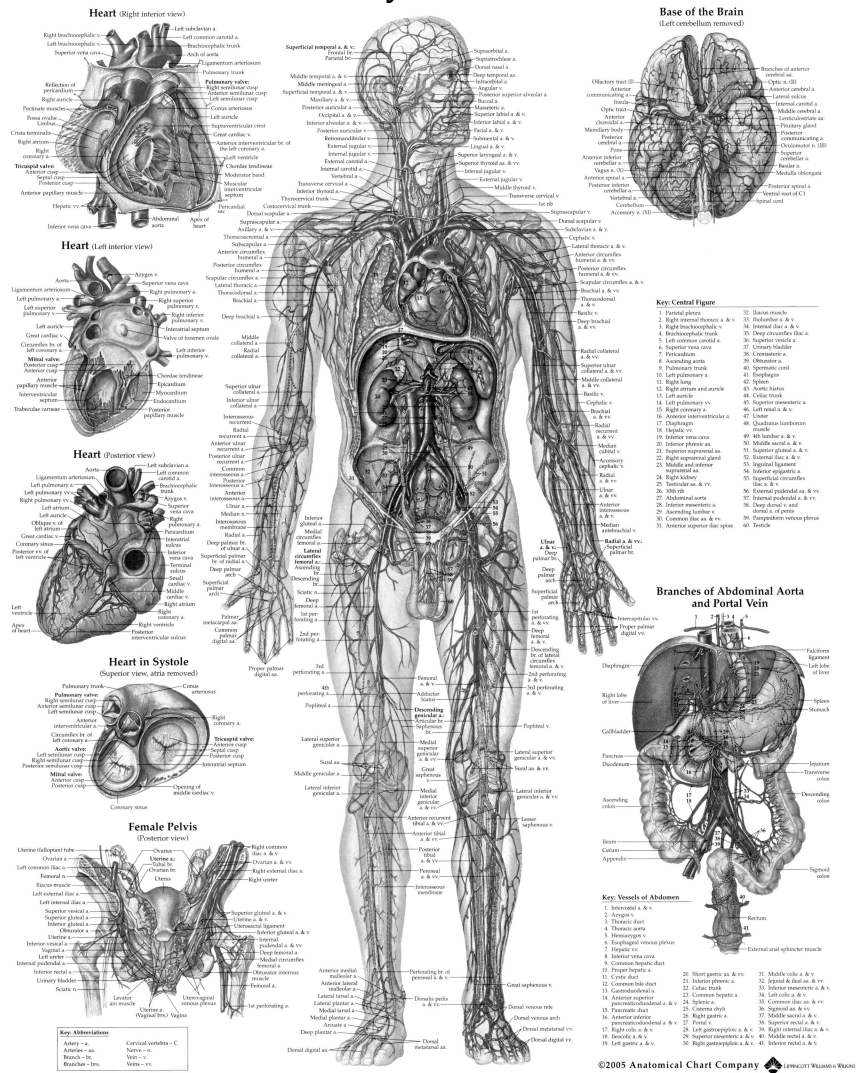

Heart (Right interior view)

Heart (Left interior view)

Heart (Posterior view)

Heart in Systole (Superior view, atria removed)

Female Pelvis (Posterior view)

Base of the Brain (Left cerebellum removed)

Branches of Abdominal Aorta and Portal Vein

Key: Central Figure

1. Parietal pleura
2. Right internal thoracic a. & v.
3. Right brachiocephalic v.
4. Brachiocephalic trunk
5. Left common carotid a.
6. Superior vena cava
7. Pericardium
8. Ascending aorta
9. Pulmonary trunk
10. Left pulmonary a.
11. Right lung
12. Right atrium and auricle
13. Left auricle
14. Left pulmonary vv.
15. Right coronary a.
16. Anterior interventricular a.
17. Diaphragm
18. Hepatic vv.
19. Inferior vena cava
20. Inferior phrenic aa.
21. Superior suprarenal aa.
22. Right suprarenal gland
23. Middle and inferior suprarenal aa.
24. Right kidney
25. Testicular aa. & vv.
26. 10th rib
27. Abdominal aorta
28. Inferior mesenteric a.
29. Ascending lumbar v.
30. Common iliac aa. & v.
31. Anterior superior iliac spine
32. Iliacus muscle
33. Iliolumbar a. & v.
34. Internal iliac a.
35. Deep circumflex iliac a.
36. Superior vesicle a.
37. Urinary bladder
38. Cremasteric a.
39. Obturator a.
40. Spermatic cord
41. Esophagus
42. Spleen
43. Aortic hiatus
44. Celiac trunk
45. Superior mesenteric a.
46. Left renal a. & v.
47. Ureter
48. Quadratus lumborum muscle
49. 4th lumbar a. & v.
50. Middle sacral a. & v.
51. Superior gluteal a. & v.
52. External iliac a.
53. Inguinal ligament
54. Inferior epigastric a.
55. Superficial circumflex iliac a. & v.
56. External pudendal aa. & vv.
57. Internal pudendal a. & vv.
58. Deep dorsal v. and dorsal a. of penis
59. Pampiniform venous plexus
60. Testicle

Key: Vessels of Abdomen

1. Intercostal a. & v.
2. Azygos v.
3. Thoracic duct
4. Thoracic aorta
5. Hemiazygos v.
6. Esophageal venous plexus
7. Hepatic vv.
8. Hepatic v.
9. Common hepatic duct
10. Proper hepatic a.
11. Cystic duct
12. Common bile duct
13. Gastroduodenal a.
14. Anterior superior pancreaticoduodenal a. & v.
15. Pancreatic duct
16. Anterior inferior pancreaticoduodenal a. & v.
17. Right colic a. & v.
18. Ileocolic a. & v.
19. Left gastric a. & v.
20. Short gastric aa. & vv.
21. Inferior phrenic a.
22. Celiac trunk
23. Common hepatic a.
24. Splenic a.
25. Cisterna chyli
26. Right gastric a.
27. Portal v.
28. Left gastroepiploic a. & v.
29. Superior mesenteric a. & v.
30. Right gastroepiploic a. & v.
31. Middle colic a. & v.
32. Jejunal & ileal aa. & vv.
33. Inferior mesenteric a. & vv.
34. Left colic a. & v.
35. Common iliac aa. & vv.
36. Sigmoid aa. & v.
37. Middle sacral a. & v.
38. Superior rectal a. & v.
39. Right internal iliac a. & v.
40. Middle rectal a. & v.
41. Inferior rectal a. & v.

Key: Abbreviations

Artery – a.	Cervical vertebra – C
Arteries – aa.	Nerve – n.
Branch – br.	Vein – v.
Branches – brs.	Veins – vv.

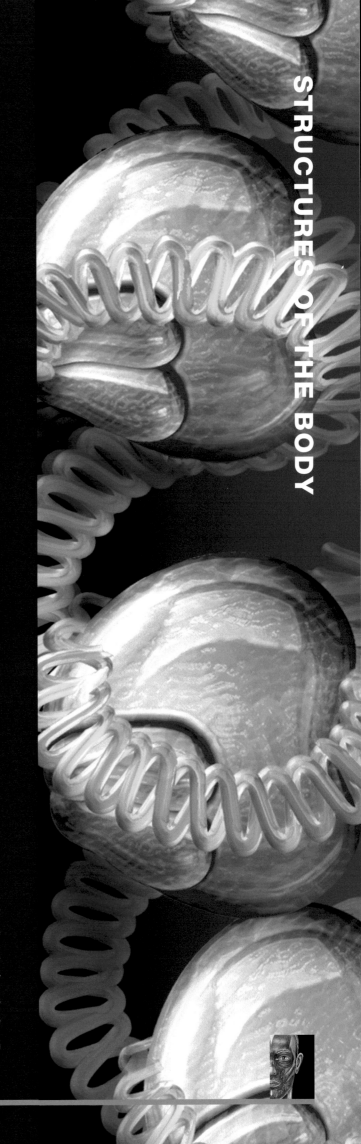

STRUCTURES OF THE BODY

The Development of Blood Cells

The Circulatory System

The human circulatory system comprises the heart, blood vessels, and blood. Pumped by the heart, blood is continuously circulated through the blood vessels, carrying vital elements to every part of the body. The blood plays an important role in transporting nutrients from the digestive tract to the body tissues. Oxygen is transported from the lungs to other cells that make up the body. Waste from cells is carried to the respiratory and excretory organs through the blood. Hormones are transported from the endocrine glands to target tissues. White blood cells participate in the body's immune system. Thus, the blood plays a vital part in cellular activities and aids in providing a favorable cellular environment.

The Development of Blood Cells

The process of blood cell formation is called **hematopoiesis**. Blood cells develop from **hemocytoblasts** (stem cells) through progressive maturation. This process initially occurs in the yolk sac, liver, and spleen during fetal development. After birth, hematopoiesis takes place in the tissue that lines the red marrow of bones. In infants, red marrow occupies the cavities of most bones. With increasing age, most of the red marrow is replaced by yellow marrow, which functions as fat storage tissue. In an adult, red marrow is found mainly in the spongy bone of the skull, sternum, clavicles, ribs, vertebrae, and pelvis.

About three million red blood cells and 120,000 white blood cells are produced every second.

The Components of Blood

Blood is made up of a liquid component (plasma) and a formed component (red blood cells, white blood cells, and platelets).

Each of the blood's components performs specific vital functions:

- **Plasma** is a clear, straw-colored fluid that carries antibodies and nutrients to tissues and carries waste away.
- **Red blood cells**, or **erythrocytes**, carry oxygen to the tissues and remove carbon dioxide from them.
- **White blood cells**, or **leukocytes**, participate in the inflammatory and immune response.
- **Platelets**, or **thrombocytes**, along with the coagulation factors in plasma, control bleeding.

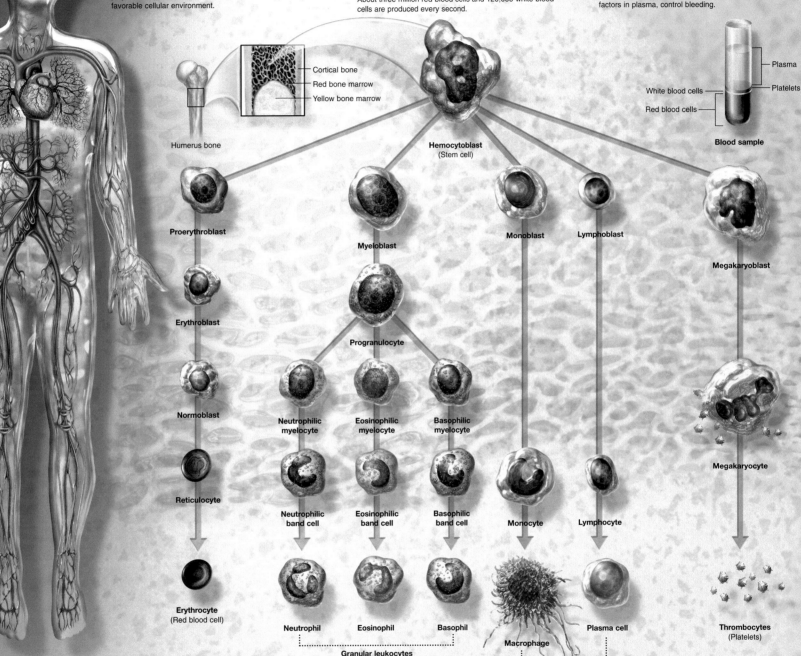

Cortical bone
Red bone marrow
Yellow bone marrow

Humerus bone

Hemocytoblast (Stem cell)

Plasma
Platelets
White blood cells
Red blood cells

Blood sample

Proerythroblast

Myeloblast

Monoblast

Lymphoblast

Megakaryoblast

Erythroblast

Progranulocyte

Normoblast

Neutrophilic myelocyte

Eosinophilic myelocyte

Basophilic myelocyte

Megakaryocyte

Reticulocyte

Neutrophilic band cell

Eosinophilic band cell

Basophilic band cell

Monocyte

Lymphocyte

Erythrocyte (Red blood cell)

Neutrophil

Eosinophil

Basophil

Macrophage

Plasma cell

Thrombocytes (Platelets)

Granular leukocytes (White blood cells)

Nongranular leukocytes (White blood cells)

Red Blood Cells

Red blood cells, or **erythrocytes**, carry oxygen to the tissues and remove carbon dioxide from them.

The production of red blood cells is called erythropoiesis. Red blood cell formation begins with a precursor stem cell called a hemocytoblast. Red blood cells in adults are usually produced in the red marrow of bone. In the fetus, the liver and spleen also participate in red blood cell production.

Development of red blood cells requires vitamin B$_{12}$, folic acid, and minerals, such as copper, cobalt, and especially iron.

Red blood cell production is regulated by the tissues' demand for oxygen and the blood cells' ability to deliver it. A lack of oxygen in the tissues (anoxia) stimulates the formation and release of erythropoietin, a hormone that activates the bone marrow to produce red blood cells. Erythropoiesis is also stimulated by androgens.

The average life span of a red blood cell is about 120 days.

White Blood Cells

White blood cells, or **leukocytes**, protect the body against harmful bacteria and infection.

Most white blood cells are produced in the red marrow of bone from a precursor stem cell called a hemocytoblast. Lymphocytes and plasma cells complete their maturation in the lymph nodes and certain other lymphoid tissues such as the spleen.

White blood cells are classified as:

- Granular leukocytes (granulocytes), such as neutrophils, eosinophils, and basophils.
- Nongranular leukocytes, such as monocytes, lymphocytes, and plasma cells.

White blood cells have a wide range of life spans; some granulocytes circulate for less than six hours, some monocytes may survive for weeks or months, and some lymphocytes last for years.

Types of white blood cells include:

- **Neutrophils**, the predominant type of granulocytes, make up about 60% of white blood cells. They surround and digest invading organisms and other foreign matter by phagocytosis.
- **Eosinophils**, minor granulocytes, defend against parasites, participate in allergic reactions, and fight lung and skin infections.
- **Basophils**, minor granulocytes, may release heparin and histamine into the blood and participate in delayed allergic reactions.
- **Monocytes**, along with neutrophils, devour invading organisms by phagocytosis; they also migrate to tissues where they develop into cells called **macrophages**, which participate in immunity.
- **Lymphocytes** occur mostly in two forms: B cells (produce antibodies) and T cells (regulate cell-mediated immunity). **Plasma cells** develop from lymphocytes in tissues, where they produce, store, and release antibodies.

Platelets

Platelets, or **thrombocytes**, are small, colorless, disk-shaped cytoplasmic cells split from megakaryocyte cells found in the red marrow of bone. The megarkaryocyte cells release cytoplasmic fragments, and as they enter the circulation, the smaller fragments become platelets. Each platelet lacks a nucleus and is less than half the size of a red blood cell. Platelets have a life span of seven to ten days.

In a complex process called hemostasis, platelets, plasma, and coagulation factors interact to control bleeding. When injury occurs to the endothelium of a blood vessel, the platelets are activated. They adhere to the damaged blood vessel and to other platelets to form a plug. Along with plasma, platelets provide materials that contribute to the blood coagulation process.

Anatomy of the Brain

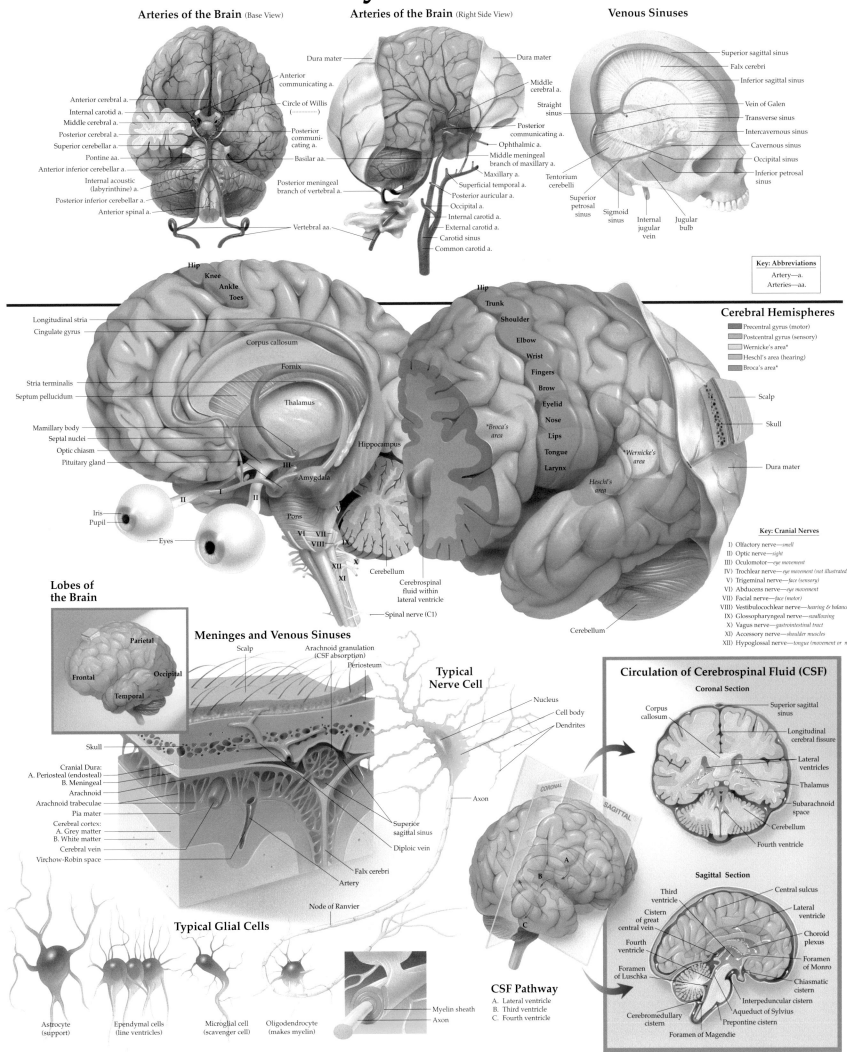

Arteries of the Brain (Base View)

- Dura mater
- Anterior communicating a.
- Circle of Willis (············)
- Anterior cerebral a.
- Internal carotid a.
- Middle cerebral a.
- Posterior cerebral a.
- Superior cerebellar a.
- Pontine aa.
- Anterior inferior cerebellar a.
- Internal acoustic (labyrinthine) a.
- Posterior inferior cerebellar a.
- Anterior spinal a.
- Basilar aa.
- Posterior communicating a.
- Posterior meningeal branch of vertebral a.
- Vertebral aa.

Arteries of the Brain (Right Side View)

- Dura mater
- Middle cerebral a.
- Straight sinus
- Posterior communicating a.
- Ophthalmic a.
- Middle meningeal branch of maxillary a.
- Maxillary a.
- Superficial temporal a.
- Posterior auricular a.
- Occipital a.
- Internal carotid a.
- External carotid a.
- Carotid sinus
- Common carotid a.

Venous Sinuses

- Superior sagittal sinus
- Falx cerebri
- Inferior sagittal sinus
- Vein of Galen
- Transverse sinus
- Intercavernous sinus
- Cavernous sinus
- Occipital sinus
- Inferior petrosal sinus
- Tentorium cerebelli
- Superior petrosal sinus
- Sigmoid sinus
- Internal jugular vein
- Jugular bulb

Key: Abbreviations
Artery—a.
Arteries—aa.

- Hip
- Knee
- Ankle
- Toes
- Longitudinal stria
- Cingulate gyrus
- Corpus callosum
- Fornix
- Stria terminalis
- Septum pellucidum
- Thalamus
- Mamillary body
- Septal nuclei
- Optic chiasm
- Pituitary gland
- Hippocampus
- III
- Amygdala
- I
- II
- II
- Iris
- Pupil
- Eyes
- Pons
- VI VII
- VIII
- IX
- V
- X
- XII
- XI
- Cerebellum
- Cerebrospinal fluid within lateral ventricle
- Spinal nerve (C1)

- Hip
- Trunk
- Shoulder
- Elbow
- Wrist
- Fingers
- Brow
- Eyelid
- Nose
- Lips
- Tongue
- Larynx
- *Broca's area*
- *Wernicke's area*
- *Heschl's area*
- Scalp
- Skull
- Dura mater
- Cerebellum

Cerebral Hemispheres

- Precentral gyrus (motor)
- Postcentral gyrus (sensory)
- Wernicke's area*
- Heschl's area (hearing)
- Broca's area*

Key: Cranial Nerves

I) Olfactory nerve—*smell*
II) Optic nerve—*sight*
III) Oculomotor—*eye movement*
IV) Trochlear nerve—*eye movement (not illustrated)*
V) Trigeminal nerve—*face (sensory)*
VI) Abducens nerve—*eye movement*
VII) Facial nerve—*face (motor)*
VIII) Vestibulocochlear nerve—*hearing & balance*
IX) Glossopharyngeal nerve—*swallowing*
X) Vagus nerve—*gastrointestinal tract*
XI) Accessory nerve—*shoulder muscles*
XII) Hypoglossal nerve—*tongue (movement or motor)*

Lobes of the Brain

- Parietal
- Frontal
- Occipital
- Temporal

Meninges and Venous Sinuses

- Scalp
- Arachnoid granulation (CSF absorption)
- Periosteum
- Skull
- Cranial Dura:
  - A. Periosteal (endosteal)
  - B. Meningeal
- Arachnoid
- Arachnoid trabeculae
- Pia mater
- Cerebral cortex:
  - A. Grey matter
  - B. White matter
- Cerebral vein
- Virchow-Robin space
- Superior sagittal sinus
- Diploic vein
- Falx cerebri
- Artery
- Node of Ranvier

Typical Nerve Cell

- Nucleus
- Cell body
- Dendrites
- Axon

Typical Glial Cells

- Astrocyte (support)
- Ependymal cells (line ventricles)
- Microglial cell (scavenger cell)
- Oligodendrocyte (makes myelin)
- Myelin sheath
- Axon

CSF Pathway

A. Lateral ventricle
B. Third ventricle
C. Fourth ventricle

Circulation of Cerebrospinal Fluid (CSF)

Coronal Section

- Corpus callosum
- Superior sagittal sinus
- Longitudinal cerebral fissure
- Lateral ventricles
- Thalamus
- Subarachnoid space
- Cerebellum
- Fourth ventricle

Sagittal Section

- Third ventricle
- Central sulcus
- Lateral ventricle
- Cistern of great central vein
- Choroid plexus
- Fourth ventricle
- Foramen of Monro
- Foramen of Luschka
- Chiasmatic cistern
- Interpeduncular cistern
- Aqueduct of Sylvius
- Cerebromedullary cistern
- Prepontine cistern
- Foramen of Magendie

*These language areas are located on the left cerebral hemisphere in greater than 90% of the population.

Dermatomes

Cutaneous Areas of Peripheral Nerve Innervation*

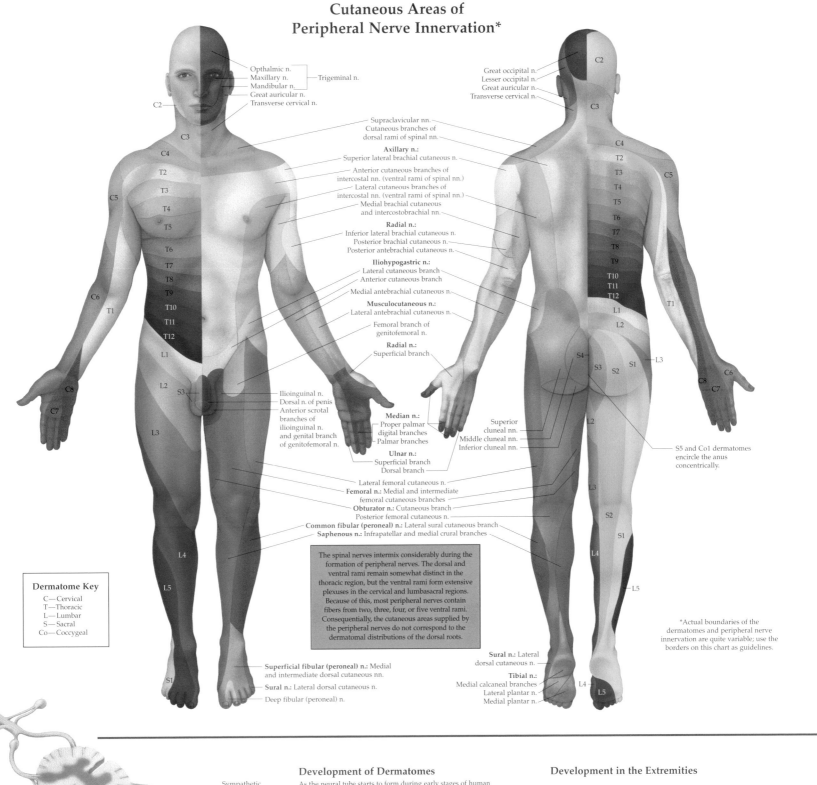

Opthalmic n.
Maxillary n. — Trigeminal n.
Mandibular n.
Great auricular n.
Transverse cervical n.

C2

C3

C4

T2

T3

C5

T4

T5

T6

T7

T8

T9

T10

T11

T12

C6

T1

L1

L2

S3

C8

C7

L3

L4

L5

S1

Great occipital n.
Lesser occipital n.
Great auricular n.
Transverse cervical n.

C2

C3

C4

T2

T3

T4

T5

C5

T6

T7

T8

T9

T10
T11
T12

T1

L1

L2

S4
S3 S2 S1 L3

C8
C7

C6

L2

L3

S2

S1

L4

L5

L4
L5

Supraclavicular nn.
Cutaneous branches of
dorsal rami of spinal nn.

Axillary n.:
Superior lateral brachial cutaneous n.
Anterior cutaneous branches of
intercostal nn. (ventral rami of spinal nn.)
Lateral cutaneous branches of
intercostal nn. (ventral rami of spinal nn.)
Medial brachial cutaneous
and intercostobrachial nn.

Radial n.:
Inferior lateral brachial cutaneous n.
Posterior brachial cutaneous n.
Posterior antebrachial cutaneous n.

Iliohypogastric n.:
Lateral cutaneous branch
Anterior cutaneous branch

Medial antebrachial cutaneous n.

Musculocutaneous n.:
Lateral antebrachial cutaneous n.

Femoral branch of
genitofemoral n.

Radial n.:
Superficial branch

Ilioinguinal n.
Dorsal n. of penis
Anterior scrotal
branches of
ilioinguinal n.
and genital branch
of genitofemoral n.

Median n.:
Proper palmar
digital branches
Palmar branches

Ulnar n.:
Superficial branch
Dorsal branch

Superior
cluneal nn.
Middle cluneal nn.
Inferior cluneal nn.

S5 and Co1 dermatomes
encircle the anus
concentrically.

Lateral femoral cutaneous n.
Femoral n.: Medial and intermediate
femoral cutaneous branches
Obturator n.: Cutaneous branch
Posterior femoral cutaneous n.
Common fibular (peroneal) n.: Lateral sural cutaneous branch
Saphenous n.: Infrapatellar and medial crural branches

Dermatome Key

C—Cervical
T—Thoracic
L—Lumbar
S—Sacral
Co—Coccygeal

The spinal nerves intermix considerably during the
formation of peripheral nerves. The dorsal and
ventral rami remain somewhat distinct in the
thoracic region, but the ventral rami form extensive
plexuses in the cervical and lumbasacral regions.
Because of this, most peripheral nerves contain
fibers from two, three, four, or five ventral rami.
Consequentially, the cutaneous areas supplied by
the peripheral nerves do not correspond to the
dermatomal distributions of the dorsal roots.

*Actual boundaries of the
dermatomes and peripheral nerve
innervation are quite variable; use the
borders on this chart as guidelines.

Superficial fibular (peroneal) n.: Medial
and intermediate dorsal cutaneous nn.
Sural n.: Lateral dorsal cutaneous n.
Deep fibular (peroneal) n.

Sural n.: Lateral
dorsal cutaneous n.

Tibial n.:
Medial calcaneal branches
Lateral plantar n.
Medial plantar n.

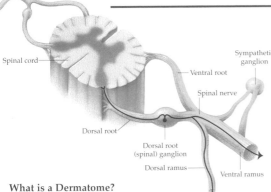

Spinal cord

Sympathetic
ganglion

Ventral root

Spinal nerve

Dorsal root

Dorsal root
(spinal) ganglion

Dorsal ramus

Ventral ramus

What is a Dermatome?

A **dermatome** is the cutaneous area (area of skin) supplied
by nerve fibers from a single dorsal root and its ganglion. Dorsal roots contain
afferent fibers, which carry sensory information from a source, such as the skin, to
the spinal cord and brain. Dorsal roots join the ventral roots to form spinal nerves at
every vertebral level of the spinal cord. From this point, nerve fibers from the dorsal
roots disperse ventrally and dorsally to supply an entire segment of skin. In the
torso, these segments, the dermatomes, form consecutive bands.

The dermatome map is an important diagnostic tool, especially concerning
disorders of the peripheral nervous system. Any condition leading to symptoms,
such as numbness, affecting specific dermatomes can be linked to the dorsal roots.
Nerve fibers from each dorsal root spread out significantly, causing the dermatomes
to overlap each other. Because most dermatomes are supplied by fibers of three or
four dorsal roots, three consecutive nerve roots have to be damaged before the
sensation of an entire dermatome is affected.

Development of Dermatomes

As the neural tube starts to form during early stages of human
development, the tissue on either side of it starts to divide into
bilateral segmented cell masses called somites. The dermatome
portion of each somite is responsible for development of the dermis
of the skin in each segment of the body. A layer of neural crest cells
above the neural tube divides in the midline and is segmented into
cell clusters near each somite. Cells from each of these clusters
migrate into the somites of the same body segment and form the
dorsal root ganglia. These form the sensory nerve fibers which
supply the structures derived from each somite.

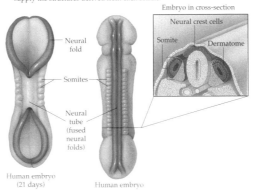

Neural
fold

Somites

Neural
tube
(fused
neural
folds)

Embryo in cross-section

Neural crest cells

Somite

Dermatome

Human embryo
(21 days)

Human embryo
(24 days)

Development in the Extremities

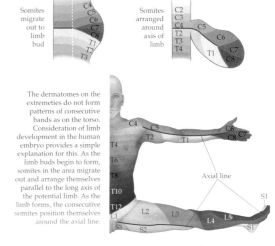

Somites
migrate
out to
limb
bud

C4
C5
C6
C7
C8
T1
T2
T3

Somites
arranged
around
axis of
limb

C2
C3
C4
C5
C6
C7
C8
T1
T2
T3
T4

The dermatomes on the
extremeties do not form
patterns of consecutive
bands as on the torso.
Consideration of limb
development in the human
embryo provides a simple
explanation for this. As the
limb buds begin to form,
somites in the area migrate
out and arrange themselves
parallel to the long axis of
the potential limb. As the
limb forms, the consecutive
somites position themselves
around the axial line.

C4
C5
C6
C7
C8

T1

T4

T6

T8

T10

T12

L1 L2

L4 L5

S3 S2 S1

Axial line

©2005 Anatomical Chart Company   LIPPINCOTT WILLIAMS & WILKINS

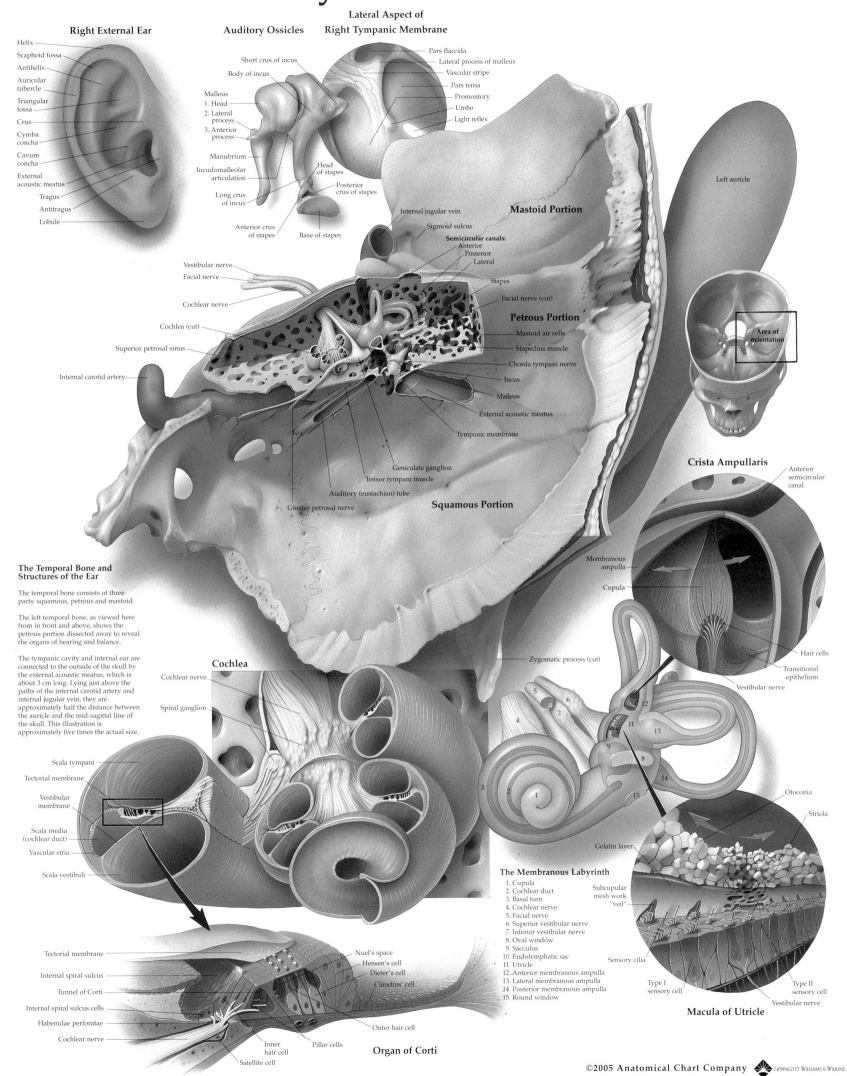

Right External Ear

Helix
Scaphoid fossa
Antihelix
Auricular tubercle
Triangular fossa
Crus
Cymba concha
Cavum concha
External acoustic meatus
Tragus
Antitragus
Lobule

Auditory Ossicles

Short crus of incus
Body of incus
Malleus
1. Head
2. Lateral process
3. Anterior process
Manubrium
Incudomalleolar articulation
Long crus of incus
Anterior crus of stapes
Head of stapes
Posterior crus of stapes
Base of stapes

Lateral Aspect of Right Tympanic Membrane

Pars flaccida
Lateral process of malleus
Vascular stripe
Pars tensa
Promontory
Umbo
Light reflex

Left auricle

Vestibular nerve
Facial nerve
Cochlear nerve
Cochlea (cut)
Superior petrosal sinus
Internal carotid artery

Internal jugular vein
Sigmoid sulcus
Semicircular canals:
Anterior
Posterior
Lateral
Stapes
Facial nerve (cut)

Mastoid Portion

Petrous Portion

Mastoid air cells
Stapedius muscle
Chorda tympani nerve
Incus
Malleus
External acoustic meatus
Tympanic membrane

Geniculate ganglion
Tensor tympani muscle
Auditory (eustachian) tube
Greater petrosal nerve

Squamous Portion

Area of orientation

Crista Ampullaris

Anterior semicircular canal
Membranous ampulla
Cupula
Hair cells
Transitional epithelium
Vestibular nerve

The Temporal Bone and Structures of the Ear

The temporal bone consists of three parts: squamous, petrous and mastoid.

The left temporal bone, as viewed here from in front and above, shows the petrous portion dissected away to reveal the organs of hearing and balance.

The tympanic cavity and internal ear are connected to the outside of the skull by the external acoustic meatus, which is about 3 cm long. Lying just above the paths of the internal carotid artery and internal jugular vein, they are approximately half the distance between the auricle and the mid-sagittal line of the skull. This illustration is approximately five times the actual size.

Cochlea

Cochlear nerve
Spiral ganglion

Zygomatic process (cut)

Scala tympani
Tectorial membrane
Vestibular membrane
Scala media (cochlear duct)
Vascular stria
Scala vestibuli

The Membranous Labyrinth
1. Cupula
2. Cochlear duct
3. Basal turn
4. Cochlear nerve
5. Facial nerve
6. Superior vestibular nerve
7. Inferior vestibular nerve
8. Oval window
9. Sacculus
10. Endolymphatic sac
11. Utricle
12. Anterior membranous ampulla
13. Lateral membranous ampulla
14. Posterior membranous ampulla
15. Round window

Tectorial membrane
Internal spiral sulcus
Tunnel of Corti
Internal spiral sulcus cells
Habenulae perforatae
Cochlear nerve

Nuel's space
Hensen's cell
Dieter's cell
Claudius' cell
Outer hair cell
Inner hair cell
Pillar cells
Satellite cell

Organ of Corti

Otoconia
Striola
Gelatin layer
Subcupular mesh work "veil"
Sensory cilia
Type I sensory cell
Type II sensory cell
Vestibular nerve

Macula of Utricle

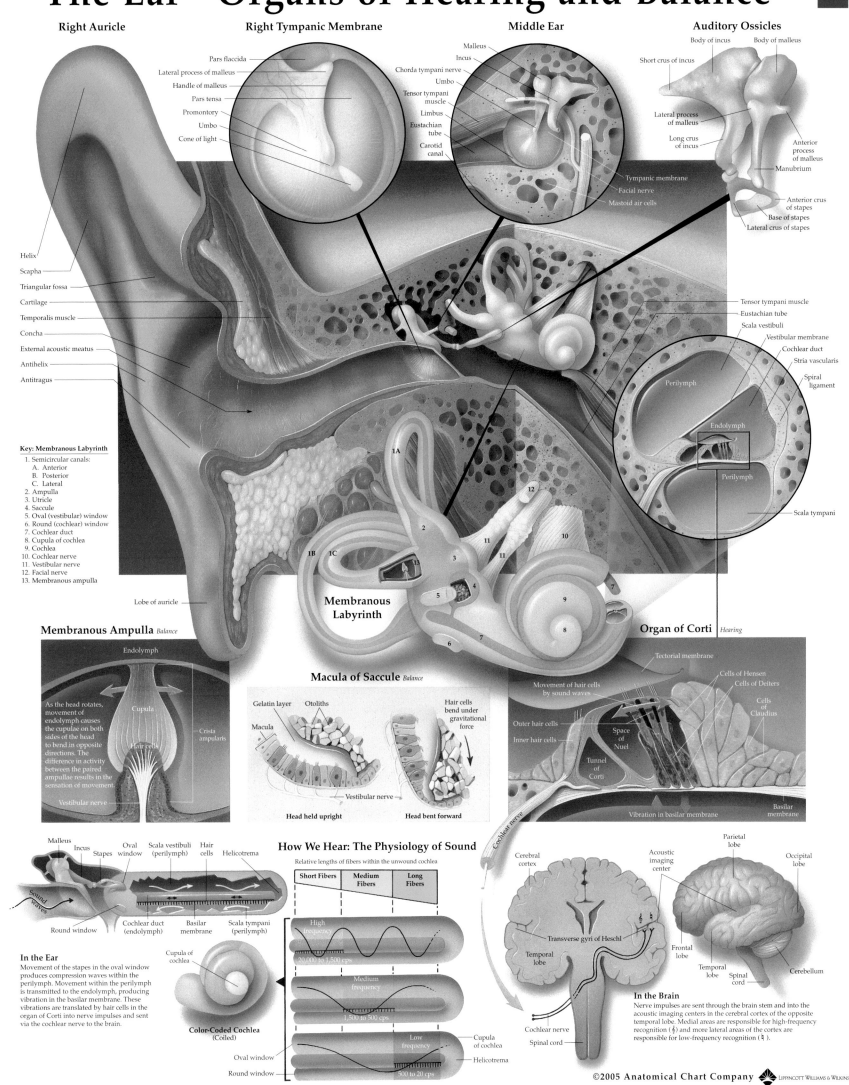

Right Auricle

- Helix
- Scapha
- Triangular fossa
- Cartilage
- Temporalis muscle
- Concha
- External acoustic meatus
- Antihelix
- Antitragus
- Lobe of auricle

Right Tympanic Membrane

- Pars flaccida
- Lateral process of malleus
- Handle of malleus
- Pars tensa
- Promontory
- Umbo
- Cone of light

Middle Ear

- Malleus
- Incus
- Chorda tympani nerve
- Umbo
- Tensor tympani muscle
- Limbus
- Eustachian tube
- Carotid canal
- Tympanic membrane
- Facial nerve
- Mastoid air cells

Auditory Ossicles

- Body of incus
- Body of malleus
- Short crus of incus
- Lateral process of malleus
- Long crus of incus
- Anterior process of malleus
- Manubrium
- Anterior crus of stapes
- Base of stapes
- Lateral crus of stapes

- Tensor tympani muscle
- Eustachian tube
- Scala vestibuli
- Vestibular membrane
- Cochlear duct
- Stria vascularis
- Spiral ligament
- Perilymph
- Endolymph
- Perilymph
- Scala tympani

Key: Membranous Labyrinth
1. Semicircular canals:
   A. Anterior
   B. Posterior
   C. Lateral
2. Ampulla
3. Utricle
4. Saccule
5. Oval (vestibular) window
6. Round (cochlear) window
7. Cochlear duct
8. Cupula of cochlea
9. Cochlea
10. Cochlear nerve
11. Vestibular nerve
12. Facial nerve
13. Membranous ampulla

Membranous Labyrinth

Membranous Ampulla *Balance*

- Endolymph
- Cupula
- Crista ampularis
- Hair cells
- Vestibular nerve

As the head rotates, movement of endolymph causes the cupulae on both sides of the head to bend in opposite directions. The difference in activity between the paired ampullae results in the sensation of movement.

Macula of Saccule *Balance*

- Gelatin layer
- Otoliths
- Macula
- Hair cells bend under gravitational force
- Vestibular nerve
- **Head held upright**
- **Head bent forward**

Organ of Corti *Hearing*

- Tectorial membrane
- Cells of Hensen
- Cells of Deiters
- Cells of Claudius
- Movement of hair cells by sound waves
- Outer hair cells
- Inner hair cells
- Space of Nuel
- Tunnel of Corti
- Basilar membrane
- Vibration in basilar membrane
- Cochlear nerve

In the Ear

- Malleus
- Incus
- Stapes
- Oval window
- Scala vestibuli (perilymph)
- Hair cells
- Helicotrema
- Sound waves
- Round window
- Cochlear duct (endolymph)
- Basilar membrane
- Scala tympani (perilymph)

Movement of the stapes in the oval window produces compression waves within the perilymph. Movement within the perilymph is transmitted to the endolymph, producing vibration in the basilar membrane. These vibrations are translated by hair cells in the organ of Corti into nerve impulses and sent via the cochlear nerve to the brain.

How We Hear: The Physiology of Sound

Relative lengths of fibers within the unwound cochlea

Short Fibers	Medium Fibers	Long Fibers

- High frequency
- 20,000 to 1,500 cps
- Medium frequency
- 1,500 to 500 cps
- Low frequency
- 500 to 20 cps

Color-Coded Cochlea (Coiled)

- Cupula of cochlea
- Oval window
- Round window
- Cupula of cochlea
- Helicotrema

In the Brain

- Parietal lobe
- Occipital lobe
- Cerebral cortex
- Acoustic imaging center
- Transverse gyri of Heschl
- Temporal lobe
- Frontal lobe
- Temporal lobe
- Spinal cord
- Cerebellum
- Cochlear nerve
- Spinal cord

Nerve impulses are sent through the brain stem and into the acoustic imaging centers in the cerebral cortex of the opposite temporal lobe. Medial areas are responsible for high-frequency recognition (𝄞) and more lateral areas of the cortex are responsible for low-frequency recognition (♮).

Ear, Nose and Throat

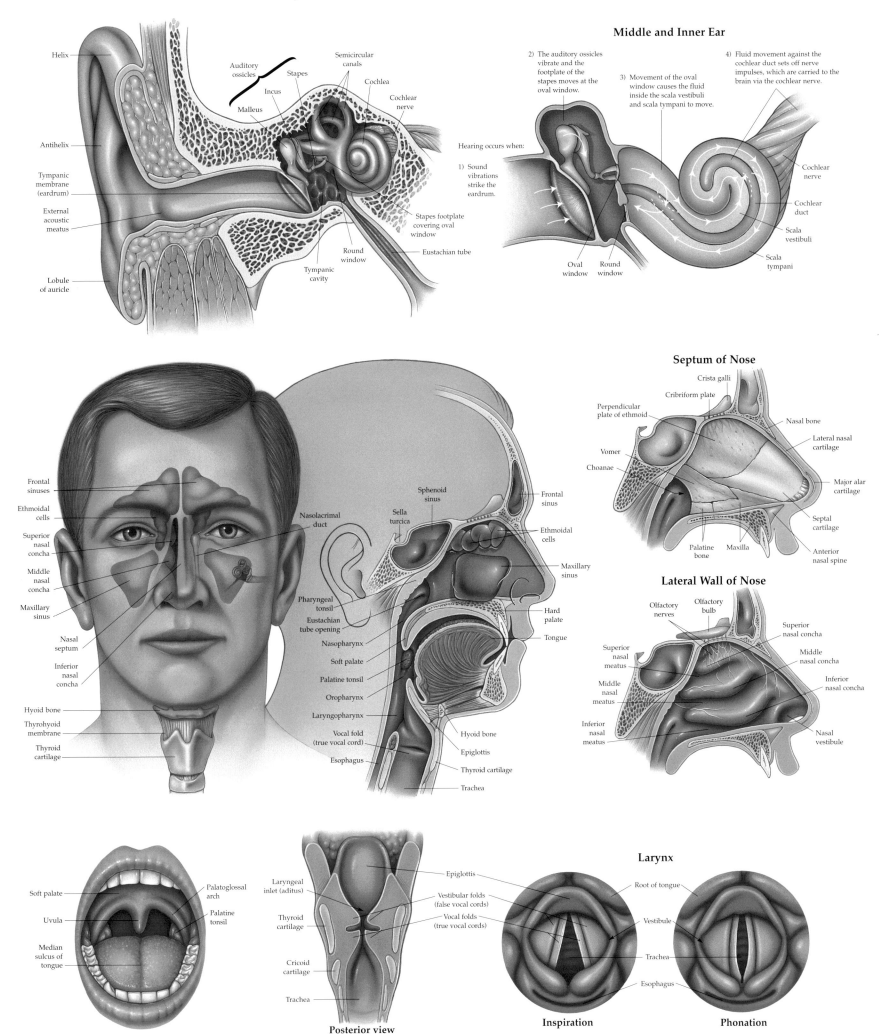

Middle and Inner Ear

Helix

Antihelix

Tympanic membrane (eardrum)

External acoustic meatus

Lobule of auricle

Auditory ossicles

Malleus

Incus

Stapes

Semicircular canals

Cochlea

Cochlear nerve

Stapes footplate covering oval window

Round window

Tympanic cavity

Eustachian tube

Hearing occurs when:

1) Sound vibrations strike the eardrum.

2) The auditory ossicles vibrate and the footplate of the stapes moves at the oval window.

3) Movement of the oval window causes the fluid inside the scala vestibuli and scala tympani to move.

4) Fluid movement against the cochlear duct sets off nerve impulses, which are carried to the brain via the cochlear nerve.

Cochlear nerve

Cochlear duct

Scala vestibuli

Scala tympani

Oval window

Round window

Septum of Nose

Crista galli

Cribriform plate

Perpendicular plate of ethmoid

Vomer

Choanae

Nasal bone

Lateral nasal cartilage

Major alar cartilage

Septal cartilage

Palatine bone

Maxilla

Anterior nasal spine

Frontal sinuses

Ethmoidal cells

Superior nasal concha

Middle nasal concha

Maxillary sinus

Nasal septum

Inferior nasal concha

Hyoid bone

Thyrohyoid membrane

Thyroid cartilage

Nasolacrimal duct

Sphenoid sinus

Sella turcica

Frontal sinus

Ethmoidal cells

Maxillary sinus

Pharyngeal tonsil

Eustachian tube opening

Nasopharynx

Soft palate

Palatine tonsil

Oropharynx

Laryngopharynx

Vocal fold (true vocal cord)

Esophagus

Hard palate

Tongue

Hyoid bone

Epiglottis

Thyroid cartilage

Trachea

Lateral Wall of Nose

Olfactory nerves

Olfactory bulb

Superior nasal concha

Superior nasal meatus

Middle nasal meatus

Inferior nasal meatus

Middle nasal concha

Inferior nasal concha

Nasal vestibule

Soft palate

Uvula

Median sulcus of tongue

Palatoglossal arch

Palatine tonsil

Laryngeal inlet (aditus)

Thyroid cartilage

Cricoid cartilage

Trachea

Epiglottis

Vestibular folds (false vocal cords)

Vocal folds (true vocal cords)

Posterior view

Larynx

Root of tongue

Vestibule

Trachea

Esophagus

Inspiration

Phonation

The Eye

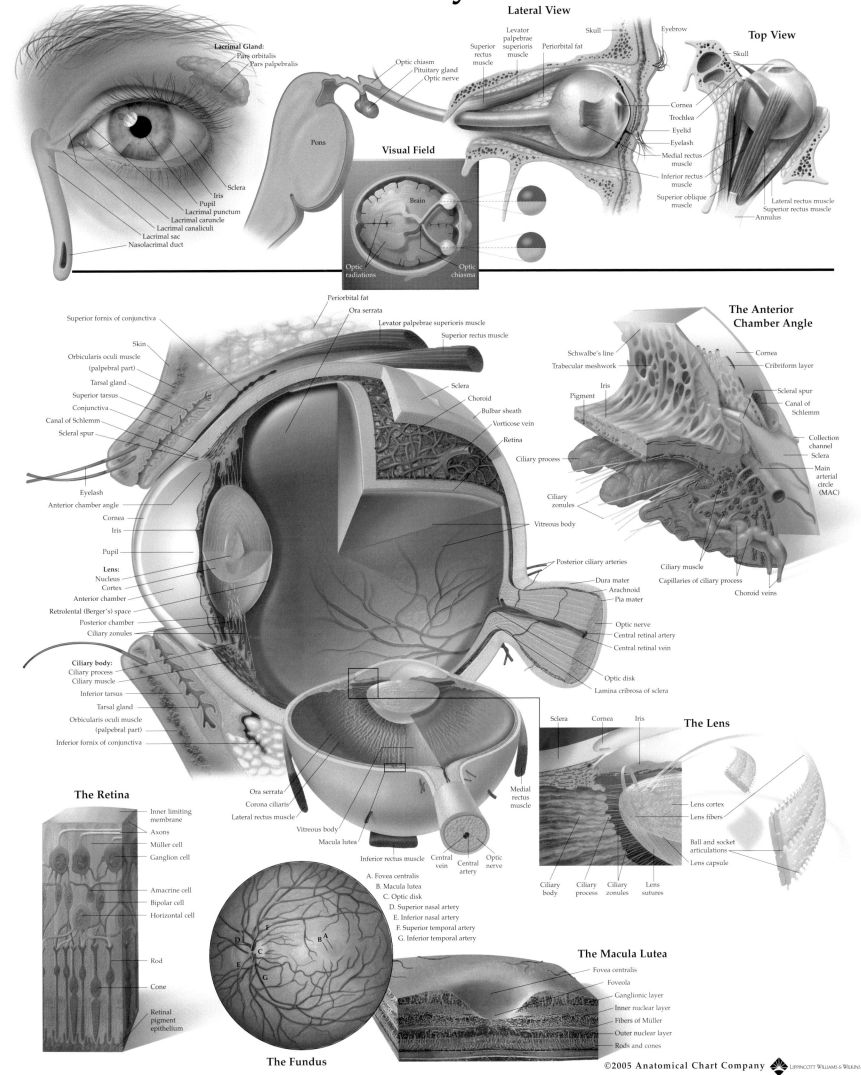

Lacrimal Gland:
Pars orbitalis
Pars palpebralis

Sclera
Iris
Pupil
Lacrimal punctum
Lacrimal caruncle
Lacrimal canaliculi
Lacrimal sac
Nasolacrimal duct

Optic chiasm
Pituitary gland
Optic nerve

Pons

Lateral View

Levator palpebrae superioris muscle
Superior rectus muscle
Skull
Eyebrow
Periorbital fat
Cornea
Trochlea
Eyelid
Eyelash
Medial rectus muscle
Inferior rectus muscle
Superior oblique muscle

Top View

Skull
Lateral rectus muscle
Superior rectus muscle
Annulus

Visual Field

Brain
Optic radiations
Optic chiasma

The Anterior Chamber Angle

Schwalbe's line
Trabecular meshwork
Iris
Pigment
Cornea
Cribriform layer
Scleral spur
Canal of Schlemm
Collection channel
Sclera
Main arterial circle (MAC)
Ciliary process
Ciliary zonules
Ciliary muscle
Capillaries of ciliary process
Choroid veins

Superior fornix of conjunctiva
Skin
Orbicularis oculi muscle (palpebral part)
Tarsal gland
Superior tarsus
Conjunctiva
Canal of Schlemm
Scleral spur
Eyelash
Anterior chamber angle
Cornea
Iris
Pupil
Lens:
Nucleus
Cortex
Anterior chamber
Retrolental (Berger's) space
Posterior chamber
Ciliary zonules
Ciliary body:
Ciliary process
Ciliary muscle
Inferior tarsus
Tarsal gland
Orbicularis oculi muscle (palpebral part)
Inferior fornix of conjunctiva

Periorbital fat
Ora serrata
Levator palpebrae superioris muscle
Superior rectus muscle
Sclera
Choroid
Bulbar sheath
Vorticose vein
Retina
Vitreous body
Posterior ciliary arteries
Dura mater
Arachnoid
Pia mater
Optic nerve
Central retinal artery
Central retinal vein
Optic disk
Lamina cribrosa of sclera

Ora serrata
Corona ciliaris
Lateral rectus muscle
Vitreous body
Macula lutea
Inferior rectus muscle
Central vein
Central artery
Optic nerve
Medial rectus muscle

The Lens

Sclera
Cornea
Iris
Lens cortex
Lens fibers
Ball and socket articulations
Lens capsule
Ciliary body
Ciliary process
Ciliary zonules
Lens sutures

The Retina

Inner limiting membrane
Axons
Müller cell
Ganglion cell
Amacrine cell
Bipolar cell
Horizontal cell
Rod
Cone
Retinal pigment epithelium

A. Fovea centralis
B. Macula lutea
C. Optic disk
D. Superior nasal artery
E. Inferior nasal artery
F. Superior temporal artery
G. Inferior temporal artery

The Fundus

The Macula Lutea

Fovea centralis
Foveola
Ganglionic layer
Inner nuclear layer
Fibers of Müller
Outer nuclear layer
Rods and cones

©2005 Anatomical Chart Company   LIPPINCOTT WILLIAMS & WILKINS

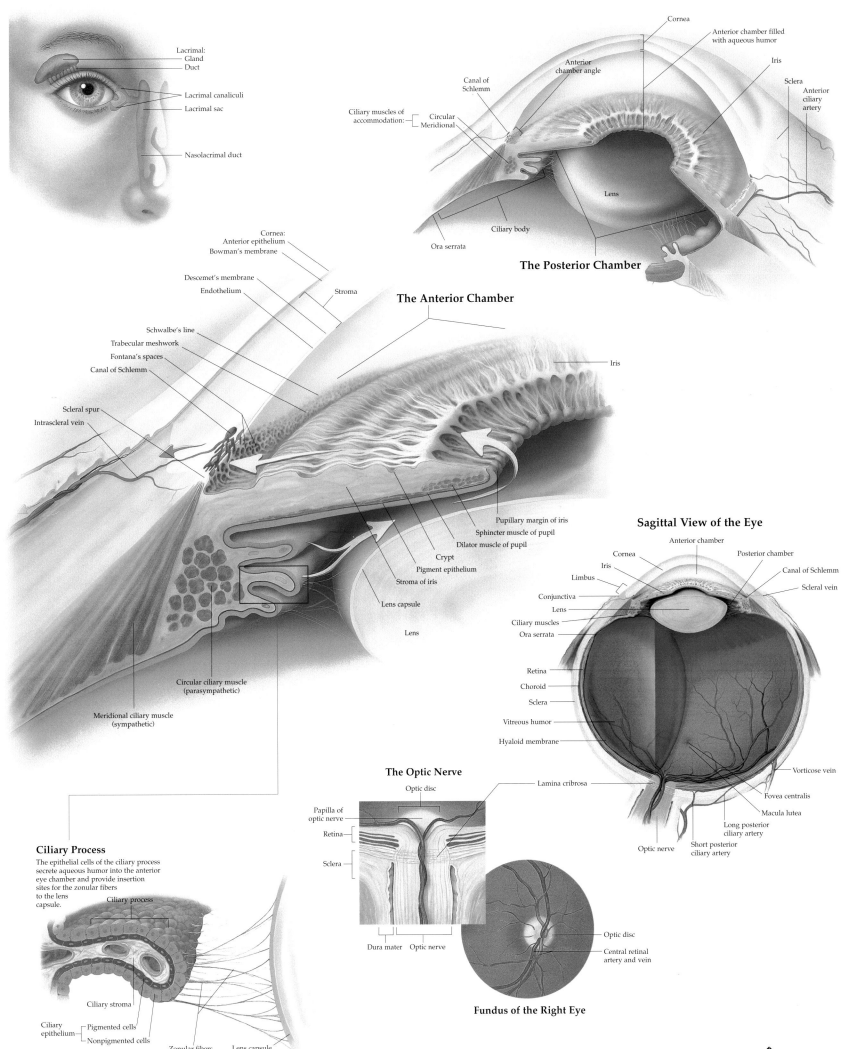

The Posterior Chamber

The Anterior Chamber

Sagittal View of the Eye

The Optic Nerve

Ciliary Process
The epithelial cells of the ciliary process secrete aqueous humor into the anterior eye chamber and provide insertion sites for the zonular fibers to the lens capsule.

Fundus of the Right Eye

Foot and Ankle

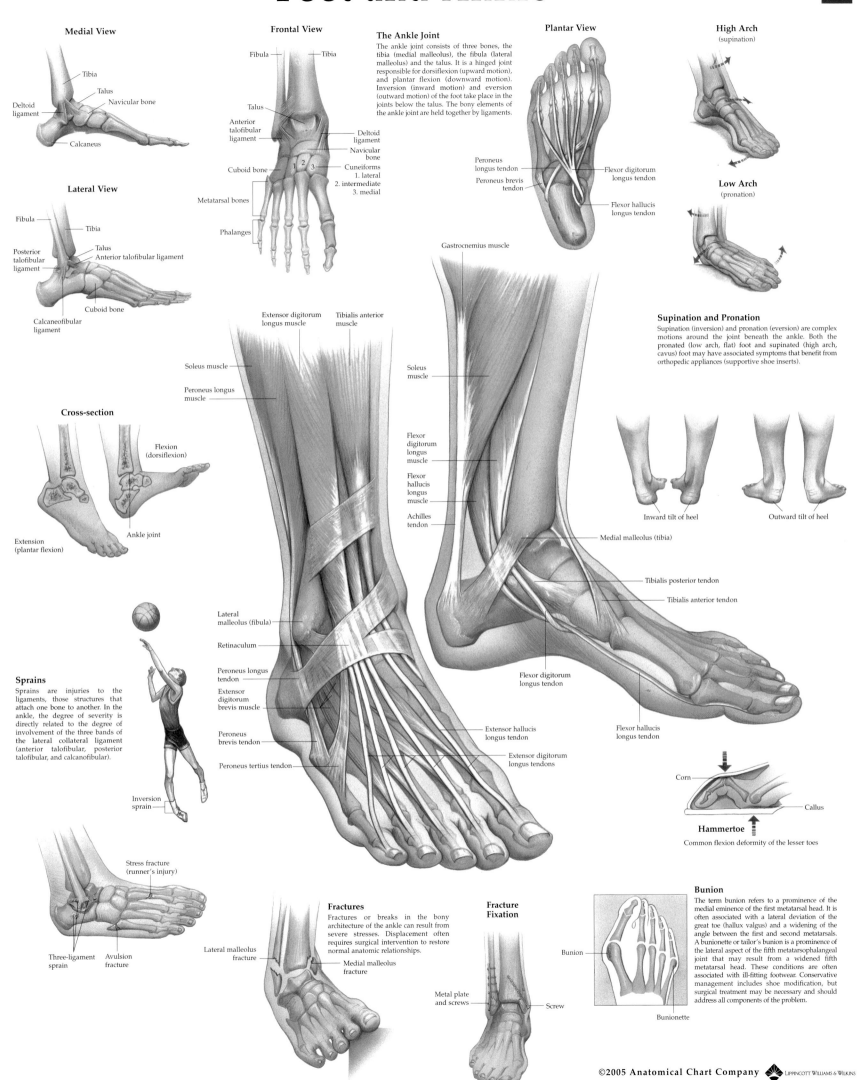

Medial View

Tibia
Talus
Deltoid ligament
Navicular bone
Calcaneus

Lateral View

Fibula
Tibia
Posterior talofibular ligament
Talus
Anterior talofibular ligament
Calcaneofibular ligament
Cuboid bone

Frontal View

Fibula
Tibia
Talus
Anterior talofibular ligament
Cuboid bone
Metatarsal bones
Phalanges
Deltoid ligament
Navicular bone
Cuneiforms
1. lateral
2. intermediate
3. medial

The Ankle Joint

The ankle joint consists of three bones, the tibia (medial malleolus), the fibula (lateral malleolus) and the talus. It is a hinged joint responsible for dorsiflexion (upward motion), and plantar flexion (downward motion). Inversion (inward motion) and eversion (outward motion) of the foot take place in the joints below the talus. The bony elements of the ankle joint are held together by ligaments.

Plantar View

Peroneus longus tendon
Peroneus brevis tendon
Flexor digitorum longus tendon
Flexor hallucis longus tendon

High Arch
(supination)

Low Arch
(pronation)

Supination and Pronation

Supination (inversion) and pronation (eversion) are complex motions around the joint beneath the ankle. Both the pronated (low arch, flat) foot and supinated (high arch, cavus) foot may have associated symptoms that benefit from orthopedic appliances (supportive shoe inserts).

Inward tilt of heel
Outward tilt of heel

Cross-section

Flexion (dorsiflexion)
Extension (plantar flexion)
Ankle joint

Extensor digitorum longus muscle
Tibialis anterior muscle
Soleus muscle
Peroneus longus muscle

Gastrocnemius muscle
Soleus muscle
Flexor digitorum longus muscle
Flexor hallucis longus muscle
Achilles tendon

Medial malleolus (tibia)
Tibialis posterior tendon
Tibialis anterior tendon
Flexor digitorum longus tendon
Flexor hallucis longus tendon

Sprains

Sprains are injuries to the ligaments, those structures that attach one bone to another. In the ankle, the degree of severity is directly related to the degree of involvement of the three bands of the lateral collateral ligament (anterior talofibular, posterior talofibular, and calcanofibular).

Inversion sprain

Lateral malleolus (fibula)
Retinaculum
Peroneus longus tendon
Extensor digitorum brevis muscle
Peroneus brevis tendon
Peroneus tertius tendon
Extensor hallucis longus tendon
Extensor digitorum longus tendons

Stress fracture (runner's injury)
Three-ligament sprain
Avulsion fracture

Corn
Callus
Hammertoe
Common flexion deformity of the lesser toes

Fractures

Fractures or breaks in the bony architecture of the ankle can result from severe stresses. Displacement often requires surgical intervention to restore normal anatomic relationships.

Lateral malleolus fracture
Medial malleolus fracture

Fracture Fixation

Metal plate and screws
Screw

Bunion

The term bunion refers to a prominence of the medial eminence of the first metatarsal head. It is often associated with a lateral deviation of the great toe (hallux valgus) and a widening of the angle between the first and second metatarsals. A bunionette or tailor's bunion is a prominence of the lateral aspect of the fifth metatarsophalangeal joint that may result from a widened fifth metatarsal head. These conditions are often associated with ill-fitting footwear. Conservative management includes shoe modification, but surgical treatment may be necessary and should address all components of the problem.

Bunion
Bunionette

LIPPINCOTT WILLIAMS & WILKINS

Hand and Wrist

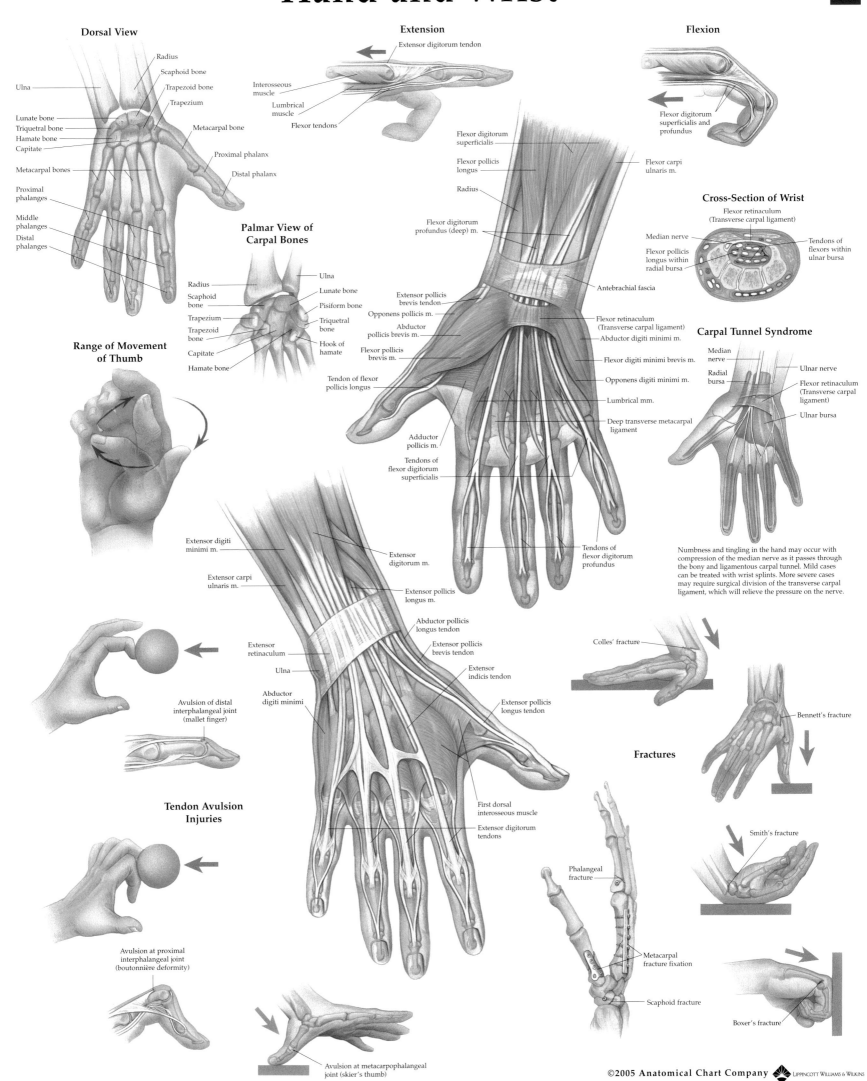

Dorsal View

Ulna
Radius
Scaphoid bone
Trapezoid bone
Trapezium
Lunate bone
Triquetral bone
Hamate bone
Capitate
Metacarpal bone
Metacarpal bones
Proximal phalanx
Distal phalanx
Proximal phalanges
Middle phalanges
Distal phalanges

Extension

Extensor digitorum tendon
Interosseous muscle
Lumbrical muscle
Flexor tendons

Flexion

Flexor digitorum superficialis and profundus

Palmar View of Carpal Bones

Radius
Ulna
Scaphoid bone
Lunate bone
Pisiform bone
Trapezium
Triquetral bone
Trapezoid bone
Hook of hamate
Capitate
Hamate bone

Range of Movement of Thumb

Flexor digitorum superficialis
Flexor pollicis longus
Flexor carpi ulnaris m.
Radius
Flexor digitorum profundus (deep) m.

Cross-Section of Wrist

Flexor retinaculum (Transverse carpal ligament)
Median nerve
Flexor pollicis longus within radial bursa
Tendons of flexors within ulnar bursa

Extensor pollicis brevis tendon
Opponens pollicis m.
Abductor pollicis brevis m.
Flexor pollicis brevis m.
Tendon of flexor pollicis longus
Antebrachial fascia
Flexor retinaculum (Transverse carpal ligament)
Abductor digiti minimi m.
Flexor digiti minimi brevis m.
Opponens digiti minimi m.
Lumbrical mm.
Deep transverse metacarpal ligament
Adductor pollicis m.
Tendons of flexor digitorum superficialis
Tendons of flexor digitorum profundus

Carpal Tunnel Syndrome

Median nerve
Radial bursa
Ulnar nerve
Flexor retinaculum (Transverse carpal ligament)
Ulnar bursa

Numbness and tingling in the hand may occur with compression of the median nerve as it passes through the bony and ligamentous carpal tunnel. Mild cases can be treated with wrist splints. More severe cases may require surgical division of the transverse carpal ligament, which will relieve the pressure on the nerve.

Extensor digiti minimi m.
Extensor digitorum m.
Extensor carpi ulnaris m.
Extensor pollicis longus m.
Abductor pollicis longus tendon
Extensor retinaculum
Extensor pollicis brevis tendon
Ulna
Extensor indicis tendon
Abductor digiti minimi
Extensor pollicis longus tendon
First dorsal interosseous muscle
Extensor digitorum tendons

Tendon Avulsion Injuries

Avulsion of distal interphalangeal joint (mallet finger)
Avulsion at proximal interphalangeal joint (boutonnière deformity)
Avulsion at metacarpophalangeal joint (skier's thumb)

Fractures

Colles' fracture
Bennett's fracture
Smith's fracture
Phalangeal fracture
Metacarpal fracture fixation
Scaphoid fracture
Boxer's fracture

LIPPINCOTT WILLIAMS & WILKINS

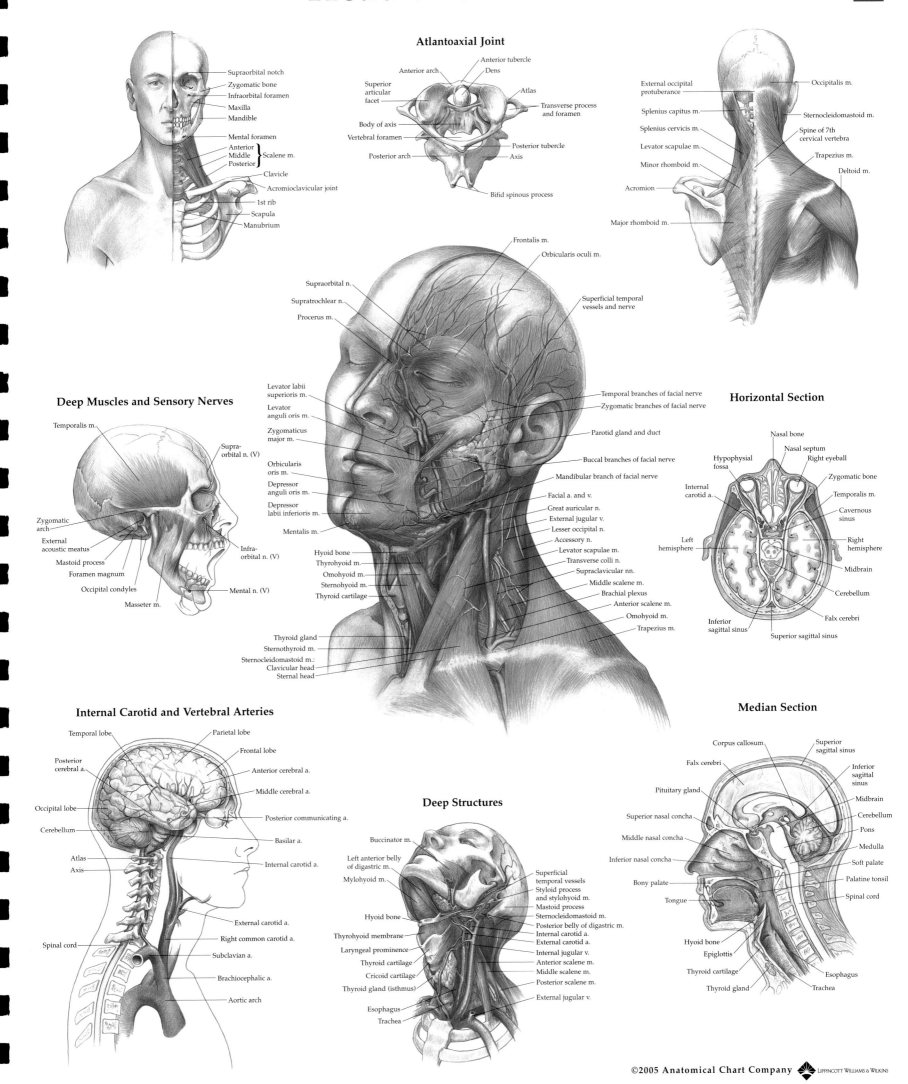

Atlantoaxial Joint

Supraorbital notch
Zygomatic bone
Infraorbital foramen
Maxilla
Mandible
Mental foramen
Anterior
Middle } Scalene m.
Posterior
Clavicle
Acromioclavicular joint
1st rib
Scapula
Manubrium

Anterior arch
Anterior tubercle
Dens
Atlas
Transverse process and foramen
Superior articular facet
Body of axis
Vertebral foramen
Posterior tubercle
Axis
Posterior arch
Bifid spinous process

External occipital protuberance
Occipitalis m.
Splenius capitus m.
Sternocleidomastoid m.
Splenius cervicis m.
Spine of 7th cervical vertebra
Levator scapulae m.
Trapezius m.
Minor rhomboid m.
Deltoid m.
Acromion
Major rhomboid m.

Frontalis m.
Orbicularis oculi m.
Supraorbital n.
Superficial temporal vessels and nerve
Supratrochlear n.
Procerus m.
Temporal branches of facial nerve
Zygomatic branches of facial nerve
Levator labii superioris m.
Parotid gland and duct
Levator anguli oris m.
Buccal branches of facial nerve
Zygomaticus major m.
Mandibular branch of facial nerve
Orbicularis oris m.
Facial a. and v.
Depressor anguli oris m.
Great auricular n.
External jugular v.
Depressor labii inferioris m.
Lesser occipital n.
Mentalis m.
Accessory n.
Hyoid bone
Levator scapulae m.
Thyrohyoid m.
Transverse colli n.
Omohyoid m.
Supraclavicular nn.
Sternohyoid m.
Middle scalene m.
Thyroid cartilage
Brachial plexus
Anterior scalene m.
Omohyoid m.
Thyroid gland
Trapezius m.
Sternothyroid m.
Sternocleidomastoid m.:
Clavicular head
Sternal head

Deep Muscles and Sensory Nerves

Temporalis m.
Supra-orbital n. (V)
Zygomatic arch
External acoustic meatus
Orbicularis oris m.
Infra-orbital n. (V)
Mastoid process
Foramen magnum
Occipital condyles
Masseter m.
Mental n. (V)

Horizontal Section

Nasal bone
Nasal septum
Right eyeball
Hypophysial fossa
Internal carotid a.
Zygomatic bone
Temporalis m.
Cavernous sinus
Left hemisphere
Right hemisphere
Midbrain
Cerebellum
Inferior sagittal sinus
Falx cerebri
Superior sagittal sinus

Internal Carotid and Vertebral Arteries

Temporal lobe
Parietal lobe
Frontal lobe
Posterior cerebral a.
Anterior cerebral a.
Middle cerebral a.
Occipital lobe
Posterior communicating a.
Cerebellum
Basilar a.
Atlas
Internal carotid a.
Axis
External carotid a.
Right common carotid a.
Spinal cord
Subclavian a.
Brachiocephalic a.
Aortic arch

Deep Structures

Buccinator m.
Left anterior belly of digastric m.
Mylohyoid m.
Superficial temporal vessels
Styloid process and stylohyoid m.
Mastoid process
Hyoid bone
Sternocleidomastoid m.
Posterior belly of digastric m.
Thyrohyoid membrane
Internal carotid a.
Laryngeal prominence
External carotid a.
Thyroid cartilage
Internal jugular v.
Cricoid cartilage
Anterior scalene m.
Thyroid gland (isthmus)
Middle scalene m.
Posterior scalene m.
Esophagus
External jugular v.
Trachea

Median Section

Corpus callosum
Superior sagittal sinus
Falx cerebri
Inferior sagittal sinus
Pituitary gland
Midbrain
Superior nasal concha
Cerebellum
Middle nasal concha
Pons
Inferior nasal concha
Medulla
Bony palate
Soft palate
Tongue
Palatine tonsil
Spinal cord
Hyoid bone
Epiglottis
Thyroid cartilage
Esophagus
Thyroid gland
Trachea

Anatomy of the Heart

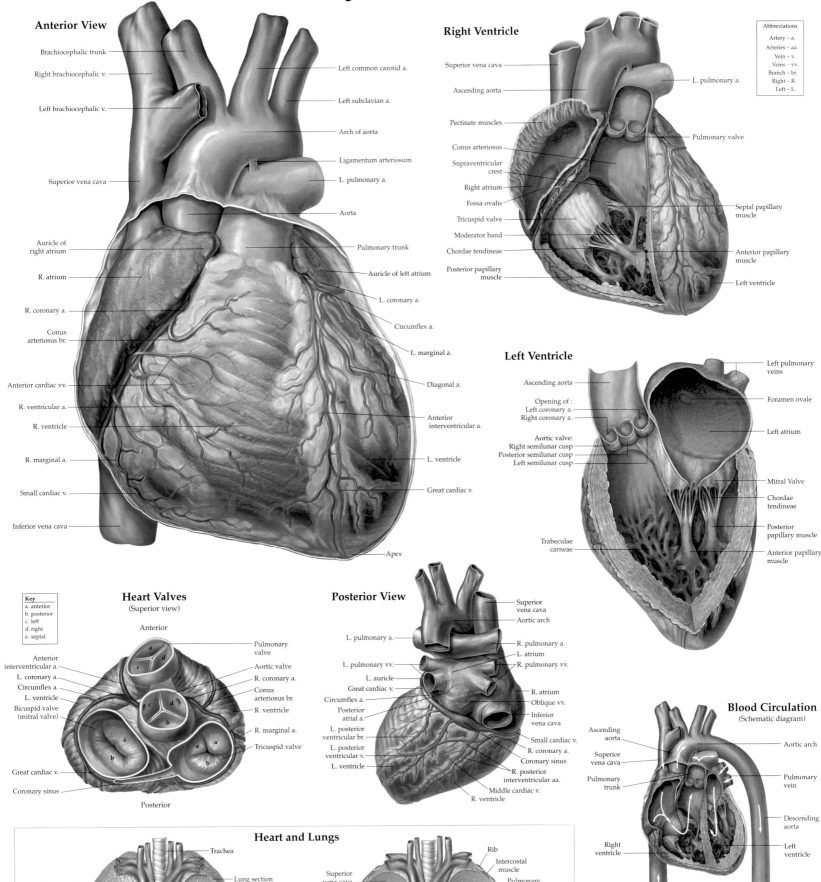

Anterior View

- Brachiocephalic trunk
- Right brachiocephalic v.
- Left brachiocephalic v.
- Superior vena cava
- Auricle of right atrium
- R. atrium
- R. coronary a.
- Conus arteriosus br.
- Anterior cardiac vv.
- R. ventricular a.
- R. ventricle
- R. marginal a.
- Small cardiac v.
- Inferior vena cava
- Left common carotid a.
- Left subclavian a.
- Arch of aorta
- Ligamentum arteriosum
- L. pulmonary a.
- Aorta
- Pulmonary trunk
- Auricle of left atrium
- L. coronary a.
- Circumflex a.
- L. marginal a.
- Diagonal a.
- Anterior interventricular a.
- L. ventricle
- Great cardiac v.
- Apex

Right Ventricle

Abbreviations
Artery – a.
Arteries – aa.
Vein – v.
Veins – vv.
Branch – br.
Right – R.
Left – L.

- Superior vena cava
- Ascending aorta
- Pectinate muscles
- Conus arteriosus
- Supraventricular crest
- Right atrium
- Fossa ovalis
- Tricuspid valve
- Moderator band
- Chordae tendineae
- Posterior papillary muscle
- L. pulmonary a.
- Pulmonary valve
- Septal papillary muscle
- Anterior papillary muscle
- Left ventricle

Left Ventricle

- Ascending aorta
- Opening of :
  - Left coronary a.
  - Right coronary a.
- Aortic valve:
  - Right semilunar cusp
  - Posterior semilunar cusp
  - Left semilunar cusp
- Trabeculae carneae
- Left pulmonary veins
- Foramen ovale
- Left atrium
- Mitral Valve
- Chordae tendineae
- Posterior papillary muscle
- Anterior papillary muscle

Heart Valves
(Superior view)

Key
a. anterior
b. posterior
c. left
d. right
e. septal

- Anterior
- Anterior interventricular a.
- L. coronary a.
- Circumflex a.
- L. ventricle
- Bicuspid valve (mitral valve)
- Great cardiac v.
- Coronary sinus
- Posterior
- Pulmonary valve
- Aortic valve
- R. coronary a.
- Conus arteriosus br.
- R. ventricle
- R. marginal a.
- Tricuspid valve

Posterior View

- Superior vena cava
- Aortic arch
- L. pulmonary a.
- L. pulmonary vv.
- L. auricle
- Great cardiac v.
- Circumflex a.
- Posterior atrial a.
- L. posterior ventricular br.
- L. posterior ventricular v.
- L. ventricle
- R. pulmonary a.
- L. atrium
- R. pulmonary vv.
- R. atrium
- Oblique vv.
- Inferior vena cava
- Small cardiac v.
- R. coronary a.
- Coronary sinus
- R. posterior interventricular aa.
- Middle cardiac v.
- R. ventricle

Blood Circulation
(Schematic diagram)

- Ascending aorta
- Superior vena cava
- Pulmonary trunk
- Right ventricle
- Inferior vena cava
- Aortic arch
- Pulmonary vein
- Descending aorta
- Left ventricle
- Capillary bed

Heart and Lungs

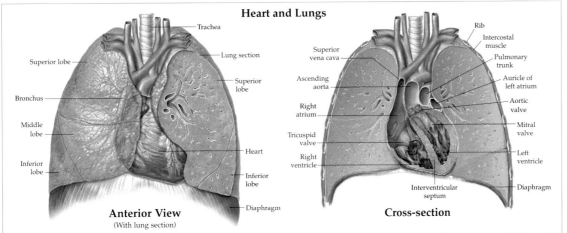

Anterior View
(With lung section)

- Trachea
- Superior lobe
- Bronchus
- Middle lobe
- Inferior lobe
- Lung section
- Superior lobe
- Heart
- Inferior lobe
- Diaphragm

Cross-section

- Rib
- Intercostal muscle
- Pulmonary trunk
- Auricle of left atrium
- Aortic valve
- Mitral valve
- Left ventricle
- Diaphragm
- Superior vena cava
- Ascending aorta
- Right atrium
- Tricuspid valve
- Right ventricle
- Interventricular septum

Blood enters the right atrium from the vena cava and flows into the right ventricle. Heart muscles contract to send blood through the pulmonary trunk to the lungs for oxygenation. Blood returns to the left atrium through the pulmonary veins and flows into the left ventricle. Heart muscles contract again to drive blood through the aorta into the arterial system of the body. As arteries become increasingly smaller, blood reaches capillary beds where oxygen is released to cells. Veins then carry oxygen-poor blood back to the vena cava.

Hip and Knee

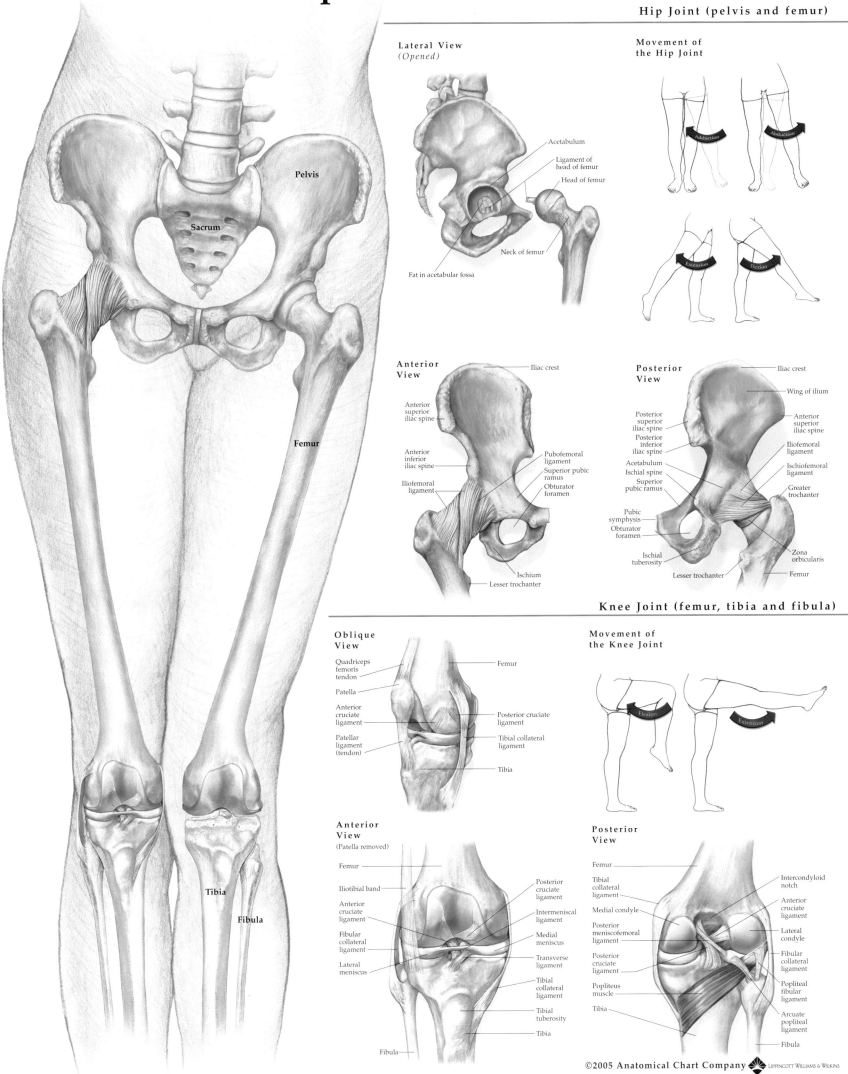

29

Hip Joint (pelvis and femur)

Pelvis

Sacrum

Femur

Tibia

Fibula

Lateral View
(Opened)

Acetabulum

Ligament of head of femur

Head of femur

Neck of femur

Fat in acetabular fossa

Movement of the Hip Joint

Adduction

Abduction

Extension

Flexion

Anterior View

Iliac crest

Anterior superior iliac spine

Anterior inferior iliac spine

Iliofemoral ligament

Pubofemoral ligament

Superior pubic ramus

Obturator foramen

Ischium

Lesser trochanter

Posterior View

Iliac crest

Wing of ilium

Posterior superior iliac spine

Posterior inferior iliac spine

Acetabulum

Ischial spine

Superior pubic ramus

Pubic symphysis

Obturator foramen

Ischial tuberosity

Lesser trochanter

Anterior superior iliac spine

Iliofemoral ligament

Ischiofemoral ligament

Greater trochanter

Zona orbicularis

Femur

Knee Joint (femur, tibia and fibula)

Oblique View

Quadriceps femoris tendon

Patella

Anterior cruciate ligament

Patellar ligament (tendon)

Femur

Posterior cruciate ligament

Tibial collateral ligament

Tibia

Movement of the Knee Joint

Flexion

Extension

Anterior View
(Patella removed)

Femur

Iliotibial band

Anterior cruciate ligament

Fibular collateral ligament

Lateral meniscus

Posterior cruciate ligament

Intermeniscal ligament

Medial meniscus

Transverse ligament

Tibial collateral ligament

Tibial tuberosity

Tibia

Fibula

Posterior View

Femur

Tibial collateral ligament

Medial condyle

Posterior meniscofemoral ligament

Posterior cruciate ligament

Popliteus muscle

Tibia

Intercondyloid notch

Anterior cruciate ligament

Lateral condyle

Fibular collateral ligament

Popliteal fibular ligament

Arcuate popliteal ligament

Fibula

30

Understanding Human DNA

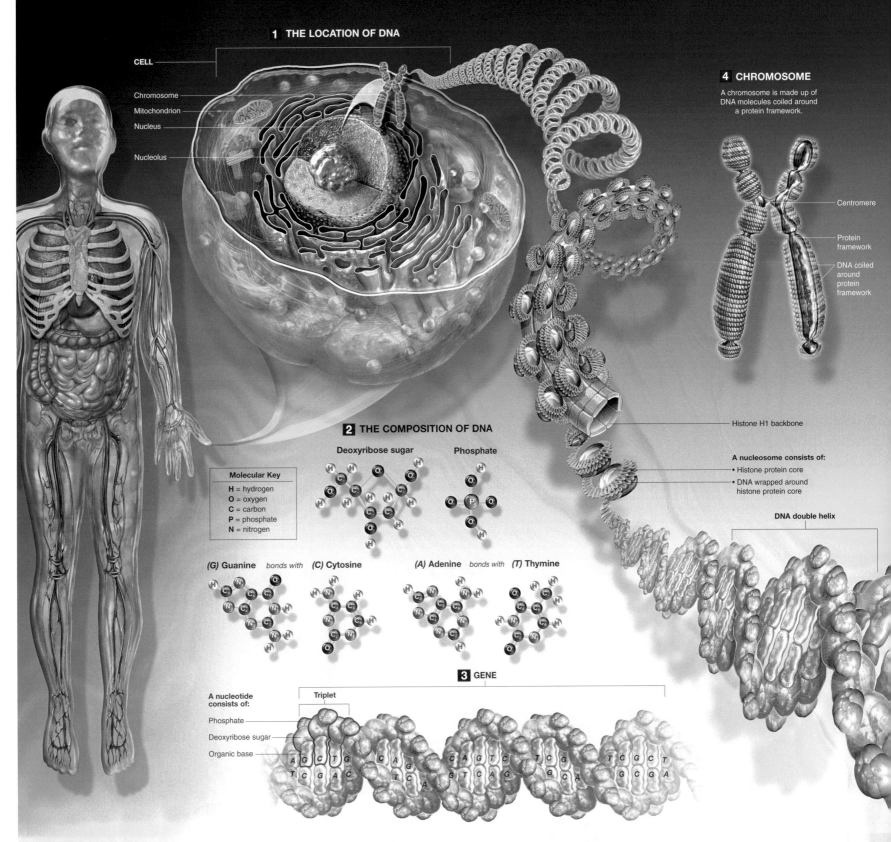

1 THE LOCATION OF DNA

CELL

Chromosome
Mitochondrion
Nucleus
Nucleolus

4 CHROMOSOME

A chromosome is made up of
DNA molecules coiled around
a protein framework.

Centromere

Protein
framework

DNA coiled
around
protein
framework

Histone H1 backbone

A nucleosome consists of:
• Histone protein core
• DNA wrapped around
  histone protein core

DNA double helix

2 THE COMPOSITION OF DNA

Deoxyribose sugar   Phosphate

Molecular Key

H = hydrogen
O = oxygen
C = carbon
P = phosphate
N = nitrogen

(G) **Guanine** *bonds with* *(C)* **Cytosine**   *(A)* **Adenine** *bonds with* *(T)* **Thymine**

3 GENE

A nucleotide
consists of: Triplet

Phosphate
Deoxyribose sugar
Organic base

A G C T G   C A G   C A G T C   T C G   T C G C T
T C G A C   G T C   G T C A G   G C A   G C G A
                    T C A

What Is DNA?

DNA (deoxyribonucleic acid) can be seen as a library containing all the genetic information that a cell needs to sustain, grow, and reproduce itself. In order to accomplish these processes, the DNA must contain the detailed specifications (blueprints) needed to synthesize the enzymes required to perform every chemical activity of a cell. If such information is missing or is inaccurate, the cell will not function properly and may even die. Thus, the DNA may be thought of as "the blueprint of life."

1 Where Is DNA found?

DNA is found principally in the nuclei and mitochondria of tissue cells. DNA can be found in two forms in the nucleus; as **chromatin** or as **chromosomes**. Chromatin is composed of uncoiled DNA strands wrapped around histone protein cores. Chromatin resembles a string with "beads." The "bead" structure is called a **nucleosome**. When a cell begins the reproductive process, the chromatin becomes more tightly coiled and is transformed into tiny, rod-shaped chromosomes.

2 What Is the Composition of DNA?

DNA is composed of two long chains of nucleic acid molecules, twisted around one another in the form of a double helix. The DNA strand is made up of building blocks called **nucleotides**, consisting of a **phosphate** group, a 5-carbon **deoxyribose sugar**, and an **organic base**. The organic base of a DNA strand can be one of four kinds: **(G) guanine**, **(C) cytosine**, **(A) adenine**, or **(T) thymine**. Because of their special molecular shapes and electrical patterns, guanine will bond only with cytosine, and adenine will bond only with thymine. The deoxyribose sugar and phosphate group are joined to form the backbone of the chain of molecules. Attached to the deoxyribose sugar of this DNA backbone are the organic bases. These organic bases are bound by weak hydrogen bonds to the bases of the second chain of DNA molecules.

A set of three consecutive nucleotides in a strand of DNA is called a **triplet** or **codon**. Each triplet contains the code for one of the 20 amino acids, the building blocks that form proteins. Sometimes, several combinations of triplets are require to design an amino acid. The sequence in each segment of DNA determines which protein is synthesized.

3 What Is a Gene?

DNA contains the genetic codes that instruct chemical compounds in the synthesis of proteins that control specific cell functions. A **gene** is a segment of a DNA molecule. The nucleotide sequence of each segment contains the genetic information for making one kind of protein molecule. Genes tell a cell how to synthesize protein molecules that function as structural materials, enzymes, and other vital substances. So genes determine a person's gender, eye color, skin color, hair color, blood type, and so forth.

4 What Is a Chromosome?

Chromosomes are located in the nucleus of a cell. A chromosome is made up of DNA molecules coiled around a protein framework. When a cell undergoes cell division, chromosomes appear as rod-shaped structures. The number of chromosomes within the cells of an organism varies among species. For example, a domestic cat's cells have 38 chromosomes, a dog's cells have 78, and human cells have 46.

What Is the Human Genome Project?

The human genome is the set of genetic information encoded in the 46 chromosomes found in the nucleus of each cell. The chromosomes are organized into 23 pairs; one chromosome of each pair is inherited from the father and one from the mother.

Thus comprising the human genome are very long DNA molecules corresponding to each chromosome. Arranged along these DNA molecules are the genes. The quest of the Human Genome Project is to determine the nucleotide sequence, the location, and the identity of each of the human genes. The task has relied on automated machines that sequence the DNA and computer programs that search for and identify genes. A rough draft of the human genome was completed in the summer of 2000.

The Human Hair

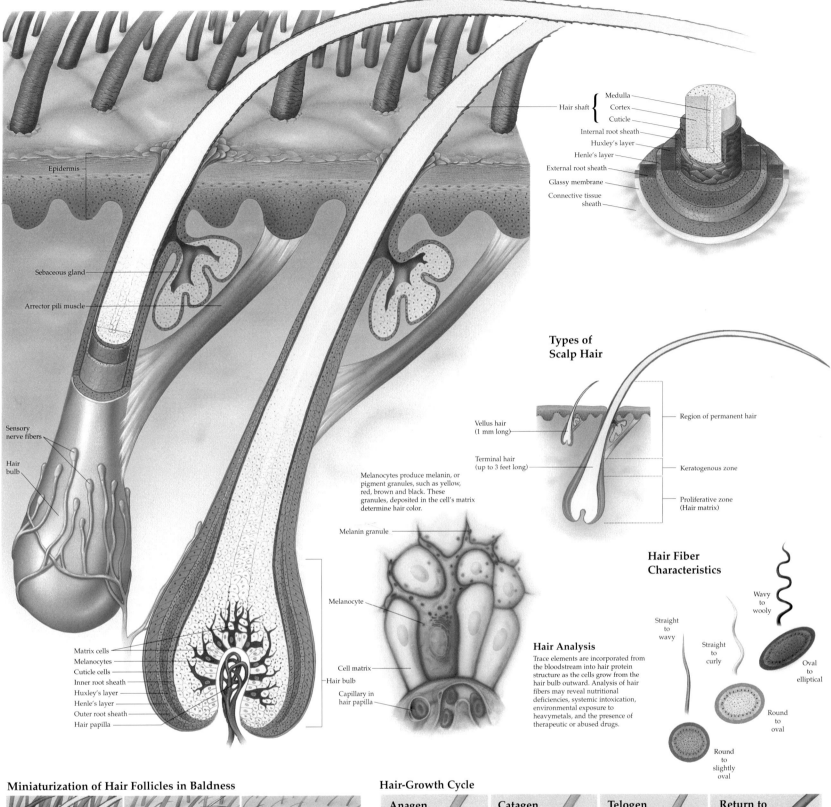

31

Hair shaft { Medulla
Cortex
Cuticle
Internal root sheath
Huxley's layer
Henle's layer
External root sheath
Glassy membrane
Connective tissue sheath

Epidermis

Sebaceous gland

Arrector pili muscle

Sensory nerve fibers

Hair bulb

Matrix cells
Melanocytes
Cuticle cells
Inner root sheath
Huxley's layer
Henle's layer
Outer root sheath
Hair papilla

Types of Scalp Hair

Vellus hair (1 mm long)

Terminal hair (up to 3 feet long)

Region of permanent hair

Keratogenous zone

Proliferative zone (Hair matrix)

Melanocytes produce melanin, or pigment granules, such as yellow, red, brown and black. These granules, deposited in the cell's matrix determine hair color.

Melanin granule

Melanocyte

Cell matrix

Hair bulb

Capillary in hair papilla

Hair Analysis

Trace elements are incorporated from the bloodstream into hair protein structure as the cells grow from the hair bulb outward. Analysis of hair fibers may reveal nutritional deficiencies, systemic intoxication, environmental exposure to heavymetals, and the presence of therapeutic or abused drugs.

Hair Fiber Characteristics

Straight to wavy

Wavy to wooly

Straight to curly

Oval to elliptical

Round to oval

Round to slightly oval

Miniaturization of Hair Follicles in Baldness

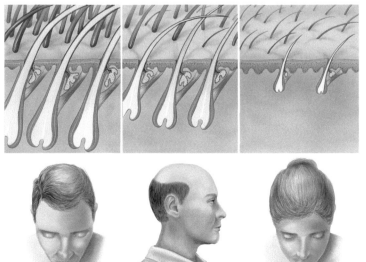

Hair-Growth Cycle

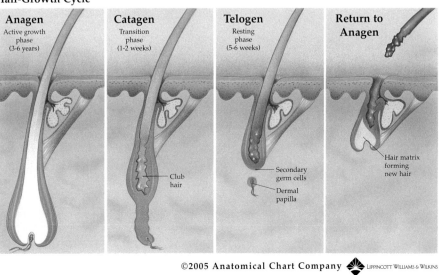

Anagen
Active growth phase
(3-6 years)

Catagen
Transition phase
(1-2 weeks)

Club hair

Telogen
Resting phase
(5-6 weeks)

Secondary germ cells

Dermal papilla

Return to Anagen

Hair matrix forming new hair

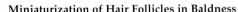

The Human Skull

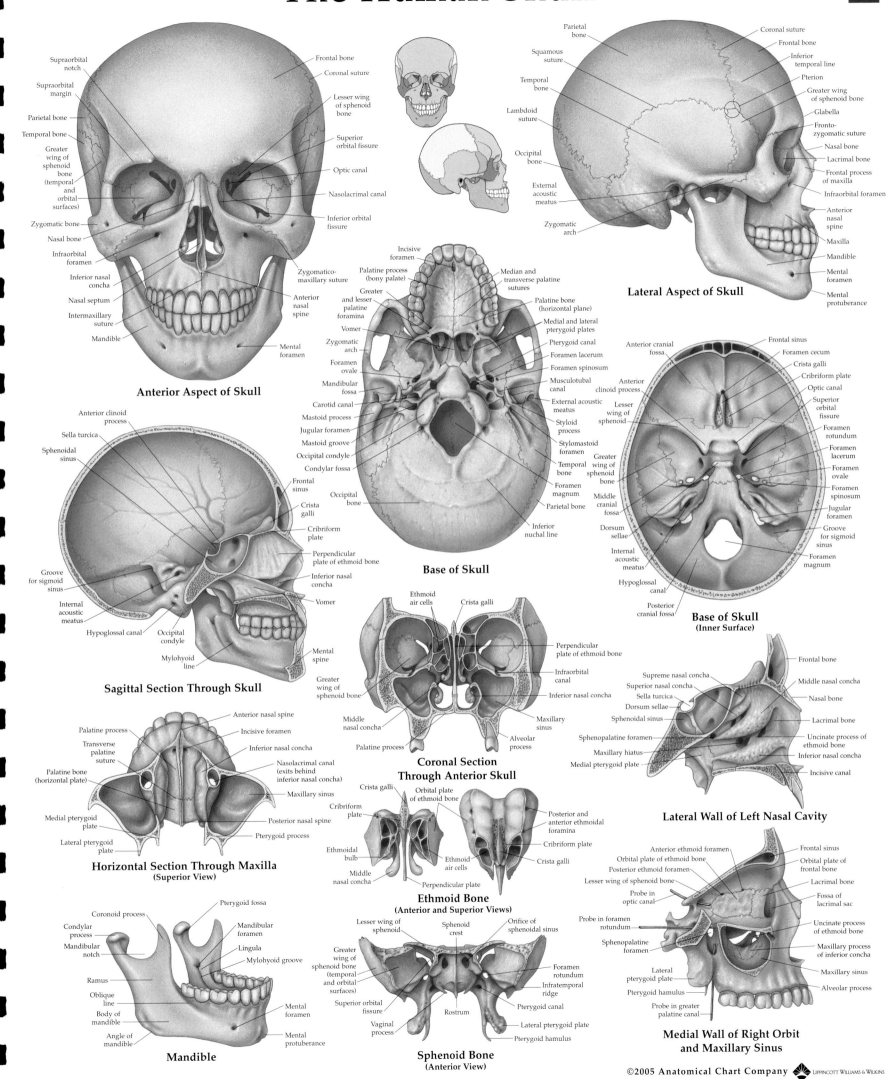

32

Anterior Aspect of Skull

Supraorbital notch · Supraorbital margin · Parietal bone · Temporal bone · Greater wing of sphenoid bone (temporal and orbital surfaces) · Zygomatic bone · Nasal bone · Infraorbital foramen · Inferior nasal concha · Nasal septum · Intermaxillary suture · Mandible · Frontal bone · Coronal suture · Lesser wing of sphenoid bone · Superior orbital fissure · Optic canal · Nasolacrimal canal · Inferior orbital fissure · Zygomatico-maxillary suture · Anterior nasal spine · Mental foramen

Lateral Aspect of Skull

Parietal bone · Squamous suture · Temporal bone · Lambdoid suture · Occipital bone · External acoustic meatus · Zygomatic arch · Coronal suture · Frontal bone · Inferior temporal line · Pterion · Greater wing of sphenoid bone · Glabella · Fronto-zygomatic suture · Nasal bone · Lacrimal bone · Frontal process of maxilla · Infraorbital foramen · Anterior nasal spine · Maxilla · Mandible · Mental foramen · Mental protuberance

Base of Skull

Incisive foramen · Palatine process (bony palate) · Greater and lesser palatine foramina · Vomer · Zygomatic arch · Foramen ovale · Mandibular fossa · Carotid canal · Mastoid process · Jugular foramen · Mastoid groove · Occipital condyle · Condylar fossa · Occipital bone · Median and transverse palatine sutures · Palatine bone (horizontal plane) · Medial and lateral pterygoid plates · Pterygoid canal · Foramen lacerum · Foramen spinosum · Musculotubal canal · External acoustic meatus · Styloid process · Stylomastoid foramen · Temporal bone · Greater wing of sphenoid bone · Foramen magnum · Parietal bone · Inferior nuchal line

Base of Skull (Inner Surface)

Anterior cranial fossa · Anterior clinoid process · Lesser wing of sphenoid · Greater wing of sphenoid bone · Middle cranial fossa · Dorsum sellae · Internal acoustic meatus · Hypoglossal canal · Posterior cranial fossa · Frontal sinus · Foramen cecum · Crista galli · Cribriform plate · Optic canal · Superior orbital fissure · Foramen rotundum · Foramen lacerum · Foramen ovale · Foramen spinosum · Jugular foramen · Groove for sigmoid sinus · Foramen magnum

Sagittal Section Through Skull

Anterior clinoid process · Sella turcica · Sphenoidal sinus · Groove for sigmoid sinus · Internal acoustic meatus · Hypoglossal canal · Occipital condyle · Mylohyoid line · Frontal sinus · Crista galli · Cribriform plate · Perpendicular plate of ethmoid bone · Inferior nasal concha · Vomer · Mental spine

Coronal Section Through Anterior Skull

Ethmoid air cells · Crista galli · Greater wing of sphenoid bone · Middle nasal concha · Palatine process · Perpendicular plate of ethmoid bone · Infraorbital canal · Inferior nasal concha · Maxillary sinus · Alveolar process

Lateral Wall of Left Nasal Cavity

Supreme nasal concha · Superior nasal concha · Sella turcica · Dorsum sellae · Sphenoidal sinus · Sphenopalatine foramen · Maxillary hiatus · Medial pterygoid plate · Frontal bone · Middle nasal concha · Nasal bone · Lacrimal bone · Uncinate process of ethmoid bone · Inferior nasal concha · Incisive canal

Horizontal Section Through Maxilla (Superior View)

Anterior nasal spine · Palatine process · Transverse palatine suture · Palatine bone (horizontal plate) · Medial pterygoid plate · Lateral pterygoid plate · Incisive foramen · Inferior nasal concha · Nasolacrimal canal (exits behind inferior nasal concha) · Maxillary sinus · Posterior nasal spine · Pterygoid process

Ethmoid Bone (Anterior and Superior Views)

Crista galli · Cribriform plate · Ethmoidal bulb · Middle nasal concha · Orbital plate of ethmoid bone · Ethmoid air cells · Perpendicular plate · Posterior and anterior ethmoidal foramina · Cribriform plate · Crista galli

Medial Wall of Right Orbit and Maxillary Sinus

Anterior ethmoid foramen · Orbital plate of ethmoid bone · Posterior ethmoid foramen · Lesser wing of sphenoid bone · Probe in optic canal · Probe in foramen rotundum · Sphenopalatine foramen · Lateral pterygoid plate · Pterygoid hamulus · Probe in greater palatine canal · Frontal sinus · Orbital plate of frontal bone · Lacrimal bone · Fossa of lacrimal sac · Uncinate process of ethmoid bone · Maxillary process of inferior concha · Maxillary sinus · Alveolar process

Mandible

Coronoid process · Condylar process · Mandibular notch · Ramus · Oblique line · Body of mandible · Angle of mandible · Pterygoid fossa · Mandibular foramen · Lingula · Mylohyoid groove · Mental foramen · Mental protuberance

Sphenoid Bone (Anterior View)

Lesser wing of sphenoid · Greater wing of sphenoid bone (temporal and orbital surfaces) · Superior orbital fissure · Vaginal process · Sphenoid crest · Orifice of sphenoidal sinus · Foramen rotundum · Infratemporal ridge · Rostrum · Lateral pterygoid plate · Pterygoid hamulus · Pterygoid canal

©2005 Anatomical Chart Company · Lippincott Williams & Wilkins

33

Internal Organs of The Human Body

The brain is the command center of the central nervous system. It receives signals that tell the body what to do and controls both voluntary and involuntary activities. The brain is the home of emotion, memory, thought, and language.

The lungs are the main component of the respiratory system. They distribute air and exchange gases, removing carbon dioxide from the blood and providing it with oxygen.

The heart pumps the body's entire volume of blood to and from the lungs (using the right ventricle and left atrium) and to and from all the organs (using the left ventricle and right atrium).

The diaphragm plays a vital role in breathing. As it contracts and flattens, it helps draw air into the lungs; as it relaxes, it helps push the air out of the lungs.

The liver, the largest internal organ performs complex and important functions related to digestion and nutrition. The liver produces bile (which helps break down food matter in the small intestine), detoxifies blood, helps regulate blood glucose levels, and produces plasma proteins.

The kidneys eliminate waste, filter blood, maintain fluid-electrolyte and acid-base balances, produce the hormone that stimulates the production of red blood cells, produce enzymes that govern blood pressure, and help activate vitamin D.

The spleen breaks down old red blood cells and selectively retains and destroys damaged or abnormal red blood cells. It also filters out bacteria and other foreign substances that enter the bloodstream. The spleen stores blood and produces cells involved in immune response.

The gallbladder stores the bile that is secreted by the liver.

The pancreas assists with the digestion of many substances such as protein, nucleic acids, starch, fats and cholesterol. Using the hormone insulin, the pancreas controls the amount of sugar stored in and released from the liver for use throughout the body.

The stomach temporarily stores food and begins the digestion process, breaking down the food with gastric acids and moving it into the small intestine.

The large intestine absorbs water, secretes mucus, and eliminates digestive waste.

The small intestine completes digestion. Food molecules are absorbed through the wall of the intestine into the circulatory system and delivered to the cells of the body.

The bladder stores urine that has been excreted from the kidney.

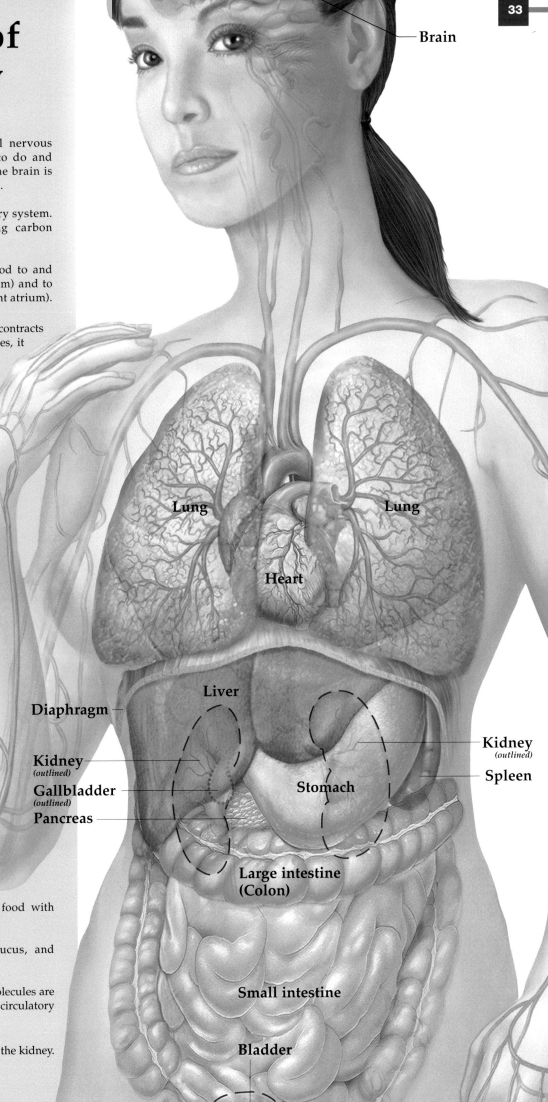

Brain

Lung

Lung

Heart

Diaphragm

Liver

Kidney
(outlined)

Gallbladder
(outlined)

Pancreas

Stomach

Kidney
(outlined)

Spleen

Large intestine
(Colon)

Small intestine

Bladder

The Kidney

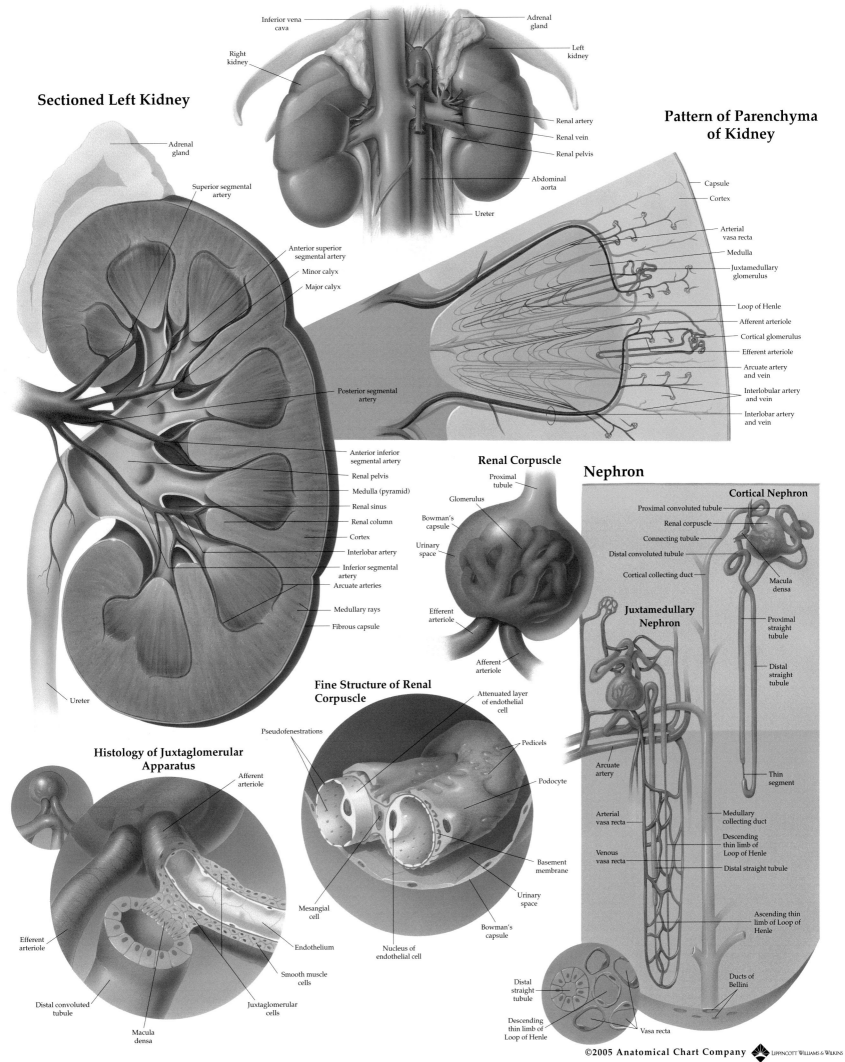

34

Inferior vena cava

Adrenal gland

Right kidney

Left kidney

Renal artery

Renal vein

Renal pelvis

Abdominal aorta

Ureter

Sectioned Left Kidney

Adrenal gland

Superior segmental artery

Anterior superior segmental artery

Minor calyx

Major calyx

Posterior segmental artery

Anterior inferior segmental artery

Renal pelvis

Medulla (pyramid)

Renal sinus

Renal column

Cortex

Interlobar artery

Inferior segmental artery

Arcuate arteries

Medullary rays

Fibrous capsule

Ureter

Pattern of Parenchyma of Kidney

Capsule

Cortex

Arterial vasa recta

Medulla

Juxtamedullary glomerulus

Loop of Henle

Afferent arteriole

Cortical glomerulus

Efferent arteriole

Arcuate artery and vein

Interlobular artery and vein

Interlobar artery and vein

Renal Corpuscle

Proximal tubule

Glomerulus

Bowman's capsule

Urinary space

Efferent arteriole

Afferent arteriole

Nephron

Cortical Nephron

Proximal convoluted tubule

Renal corpuscle

Connecting tubule

Distal convoluted tubule

Cortical collecting duct

Macula densa

Juxtamedullary Nephron

Arcuate artery

Arterial vasa recta

Venous vasa recta

Proximal straight tubule

Distal straight tubule

Thin segment

Medullary collecting duct

Descending thin limb of Loop of Henle

Distal straight tubule

Ascending thin limb of Loop of Henle

Ducts of Bellini

Distal straight tubule

Descending thin limb of Loop of Henle

Vasa recta

Fine Structure of Renal Corpuscle

Attenuated layer of endothelial cell

Pseudofenestrations

Pedicels

Podocyte

Basement membrane

Urinary space

Bowman's capsule

Mesangial cell

Endothelium

Nucleus of endothelial cell

Histology of Juxtaglomerular Apparatus

Afferent arteriole

Efferent arteriole

Distal convoluted tubule

Macula densa

Juxtaglomerular cells

Smooth muscle cells

35

Ligaments of the Joints

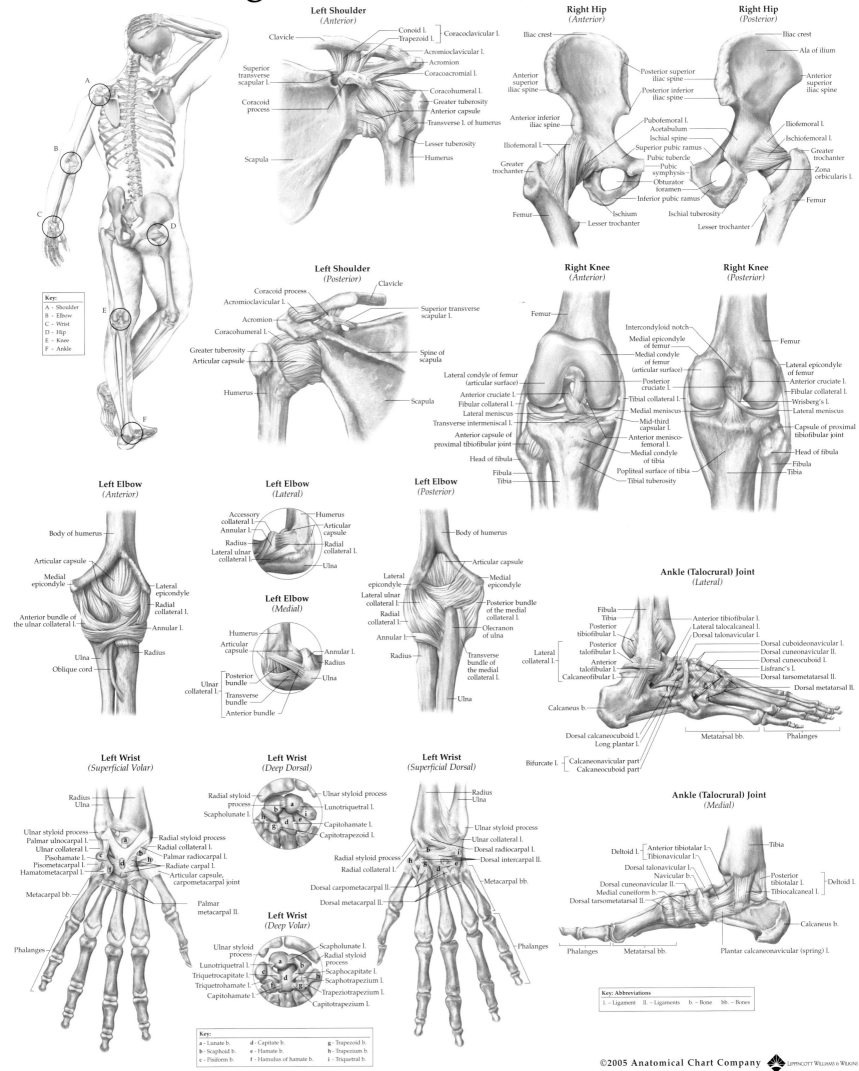

Left Shoulder *(Anterior)*

Clavicle — Conoid l. — Trapezoid l. — Coracoclavicular l. — Acromioclavicular l. — Acromion — Coracoacromial l. — Coracohumeral l. — Greater tuberosity — Anterior capsule — Transverse l. of humerus — Lesser tuberosity — Humerus — Superior transverse scapular l. — Coracoid process — Scapula

Right Hip *(Anterior)*

Iliac crest — Anterior superior iliac spine — Anterior inferior iliac spine — Iliofemoral l. — Greater trochanter — Femur — Lesser trochanter — Ischium — Inferior pubic ramus — Obturator foramen — Pubic symphysis — Pubic tubercle — Superior pubic ramus — Ischial spine — Acetabulum — Pubofemoral l. — Posterior inferior iliac spine — Posterior superior iliac spine

Right Hip *(Posterior)*

Iliac crest — Ala of ilium — Anterior superior iliac spine — Iliofemoral l. — Ischiofemoral l. — Greater trochanter — Zona orbicularis l. — Femur — Lesser trochanter — Ischial tuberosity

Left Shoulder *(Posterior)*

Coracoid process — Acromioclavicular l. — Acromion — Coracohumeral l. — Greater tuberosity — Articular capsule — Humerus — Clavicle — Superior transverse scapular l. — Spine of scapula — Scapula

Right Knee *(Anterior)*

Femur — Lateral condyle of femur (articular surface) — Anterior cruciate l. — Fibular collateral l. — Lateral meniscus — Transverse intermeniscal l. — Anterior capsule of proximal tibiofibular joint — Head of fibula — Fibula — Tibia — Intercondyloid notch — Medial epicondyle of femur — Medial condyle of femur (articular surface) — Posterior cruciate l. — Tibial collateral l. — Medial meniscus — Mid-third capsular l. — Anterior menisco-femoral l. — Medial condyle of tibia — Popliteal surface of tibia — Tibial tuberosity

Right Knee *(Posterior)*

Femur — Lateral epicondyle of femur — Anterior cruciate l. — Fibular collateral l. — Wrisberg's l. — Lateral meniscus — Capsule of proximal tibiofibular joint — Head of fibula — Fibula — Tibia

Left Elbow *(Anterior)*

Body of humerus — Articular capsule — Medial epicondyle — Anterior bundle of the ulnar collateral l. — Ulna — Oblique cord — Lateral epicondyle — Radial collateral l. — Annular l. — Radius

Left Elbow *(Lateral)*

Accessory collateral l. — Annular l. — Radius — Lateral ulnar collateral l. — Humerus — Articular capsule — Radial collateral l. — Ulna

Left Elbow *(Medial)*

Humerus — Articular capsule — Posterior bundle — Transverse bundle — Anterior bundle — Annular l. — Radius — Ulna

Left Elbow *(Posterior)*

Lateral epicondyle — Lateral ulnar collateral l. — Radial collateral l. — Annular l. — Radius — Body of humerus — Articular capsule — Medial epicondyle — Posterior bundle of the medial collateral l. — Olecranon of ulna — Transverse bundle of the medial collateral l. — Ulna

Ankle (Talocrural) Joint *(Lateral)*

Fibula — Tibia — Posterior tibiofibular l. — Lateral collateral l. — Posterior talofibular l. — Anterior talofibular l. — Calcaneofibular l. — Calcaneus b. — Dorsal calcaneocuboid l. — Long plantar l. — Bifurcate l. — Calcaneonavicular part — Calcaneocuboid part — Metatarsal bb. — Anterior tibiofibular l. — Lateral talocalcaneal l. — Dorsal talonavicular l. — Dorsal cuboideonavicular l. — Dorsal cuneonavicular ll. — Dorsal cuneocuboid l. — Lisfranc's l. — Dorsal tarsometatarsal ll. — Dorsal metatarsal ll. — Phalanges

Left Wrist *(Superficial Volar)*

Radius — Ulna — Ulnar styloid process — Palmar ulnocarpal l. — Ulnar collateral l. — Pisohamate l. — Pisometacarpal l. — Hamatometacarpal l. — Metacarpal bb. — Phalanges — Radial styloid process — Radial collateral l. — Palmar radiocarpal l. — Radiate carpal l. — Articular capsule, carpometacarpal joint — Palmar metacarpal ll.

Left Wrist *(Deep Dorsal)*

Radial styloid process — Scapholunate l. — Ulnar styloid process — Lunotriquetral l. — Capitohamate l. — Capitotrapezoid l. — a b c d e f g h i

Left Wrist *(Superficial Dorsal)*

Radius — Ulna — Ulnar styloid process — Ulnar collateral l. — Dorsal radiocarpal l. — Dorsal intercarpal l. — Metacarpal bb. — Phalanges — Radial styloid process — Radial collateral l. — Dorsal carpometacarpal ll. — Dorsal metacarpal ll.

Left Wrist *(Deep Volar)*

Ulnar styloid process — Lunotriquetral l. — Triquetrocapitate l. — Triquetrohamate l. — Capitohamate l. — Scapholunate l. — Radial styloid process — Scaphocapitate l. — Scaphotrapezium l. — Trapeziotrapezium l. — Capitotrapezium l.

Ankle (Talocrural) Joint *(Medial)*

Deltoid l. — Anterior tibiotalar l. — Tibionavicular l. — Dorsal talonavicular l. — Navicular b. — Dorsal cuneonavicular ll. — Medial cuneiform b. — Dorsal tarsometatarsal ll. — Phalanges — Metatarsal bb. — Tibia — Posterior tibiotalar l. — Tibiocalcaneal l. — Deltoid l. — Calcaneus b. — Plantar calcaneonavicular (spring) l.

Key:
A - Shoulder
B - Elbow
C - Wrist
D - Hip
E - Knee
F - Ankle

Key:
a - Lunate b.
b - Scaphoid b.
c - Pisiform b.
d - Capitate b.
e - Hamate b.
f - Hamulus of hamate b.
g - Trapezoid b.
h - Trapezium b.
i - Triquetral b.

Key: Abbreviations
l. – Ligament   ll. – Ligaments   b. – Bone   bb. – Bones

©2005 Anatomical Chart Company   LIPPINCOTT WILLIAMS & WILKINS

The Liver

36

Distribution of Vessels and Ducts

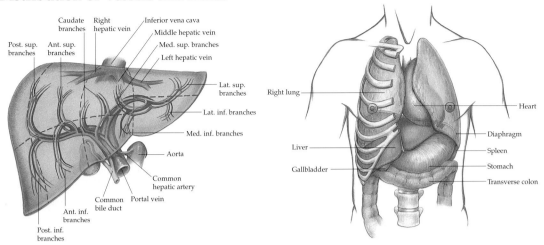

Labels: Caudate branches, Right hepatic vein, Inferior vena cava, Middle hepatic vein, Med. sup. branches, Left hepatic vein, Post. sup. branches, Ant. sup. branches, Lat. sup. branches, Lat. inf. branches, Med. inf. branches, Aorta, Common hepatic artery, Common bile duct, Portal vein, Ant. inf. branches, Post. inf. branches

Right lung, Heart, Liver, Diaphragm, Gallbladder, Spleen, Stomach, Transverse colon

Duct System with Gallstones in Common Sites

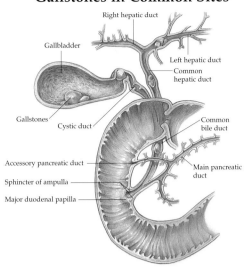

Labels: Right hepatic duct, Gallbladder, Left hepatic duct, Common hepatic duct, Gallstones, Cystic duct, Common bile duct, Accessory pancreatic duct, Main pancreatic duct, Sphincter of ampulla, Major duodenal papilla

Liver Segments Visceral View with Biliary Draining Areas

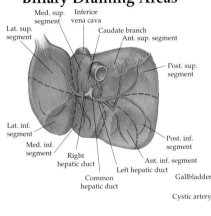

Labels: Med. sup. segment, Inferior vena cava, Lat. sup. segment, Caudate branch, Ant. sup. segment, Post. sup. segment, Lat. inf. segment, Med. inf. segment, Right hepatic duct, Left hepatic duct, Common hepatic duct, Gallbladder, Cystic artery, Post. inf. segment, Ant. inf. segment

Antero-Visceral View

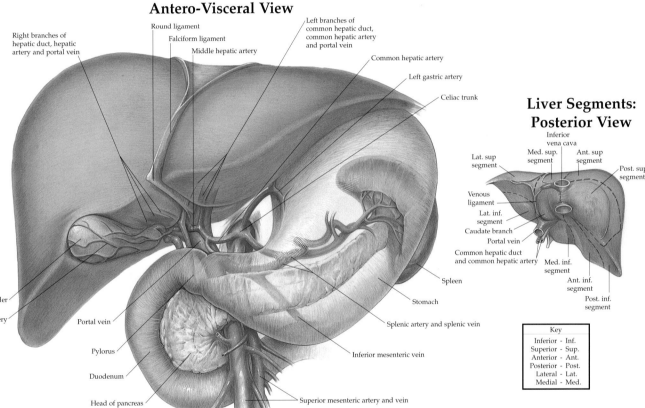

Labels: Right branches of hepatic duct, hepatic artery and portal vein, Round ligament, Falciform ligament, Middle hepatic artery, Left branches of common hepatic duct, common hepatic artery and portal vein, Common hepatic artery, Left gastric artery, Celiac trunk, Portal vein, Pylorus, Duodenum, Head of pancreas, Superior mesenteric artery and vein, Inferior mesenteric vein, Splenic artery and splenic vein, Stomach, Spleen

Key
Inferior - Inf.
Superior - Sup.
Anterior - Ant.
Posterior - Post.
Lateral - Lat.
Medial - Med.

Liver Segments: Posterior View

Labels: Inferior vena cava, Med. sup. segment, Ant. sup. segment, Lat. sup. segment, Post. sup. segment, Venous ligament, Lat. inf. segment, Caudate branch, Portal vein, Common hepatic duct and common hepatic artery, Med. inf. segment, Ant. inf. segment, Post. inf. segment

Portal System

Labels: Right branch of portal vein, Left branch of portal vein, Portal vein, Right and left gastric veins, Splenic vein, Right and left gastroepiploic veins, Superior mesenteric vein, Inferior mesenteric vein, Inferior pancreatico-duodenal vein

Liver Lobule

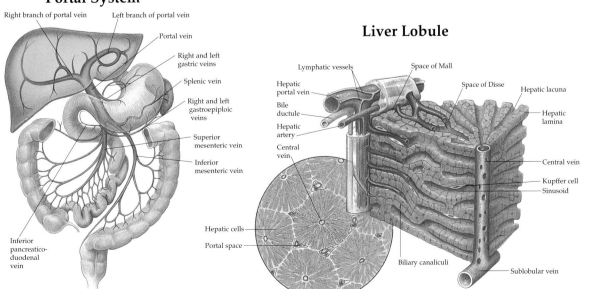

Labels: Lymphatic vessels, Space of Mall, Hepatic portal vein, Space of Disse, Hepatic lacuna, Bile ductule, Hepatic artery, Hepatic lamina, Central vein, Central vein, Kupffer cell, Sinusoid, Hepatic cells, Portal space, Biliary canaliculi, Sublobular vein

Cirrhosis

Labels: Fibrous septa, Regenerative nodules, Fatty cyst, Fibrous septa, Regenerative nodule, Necrotic area

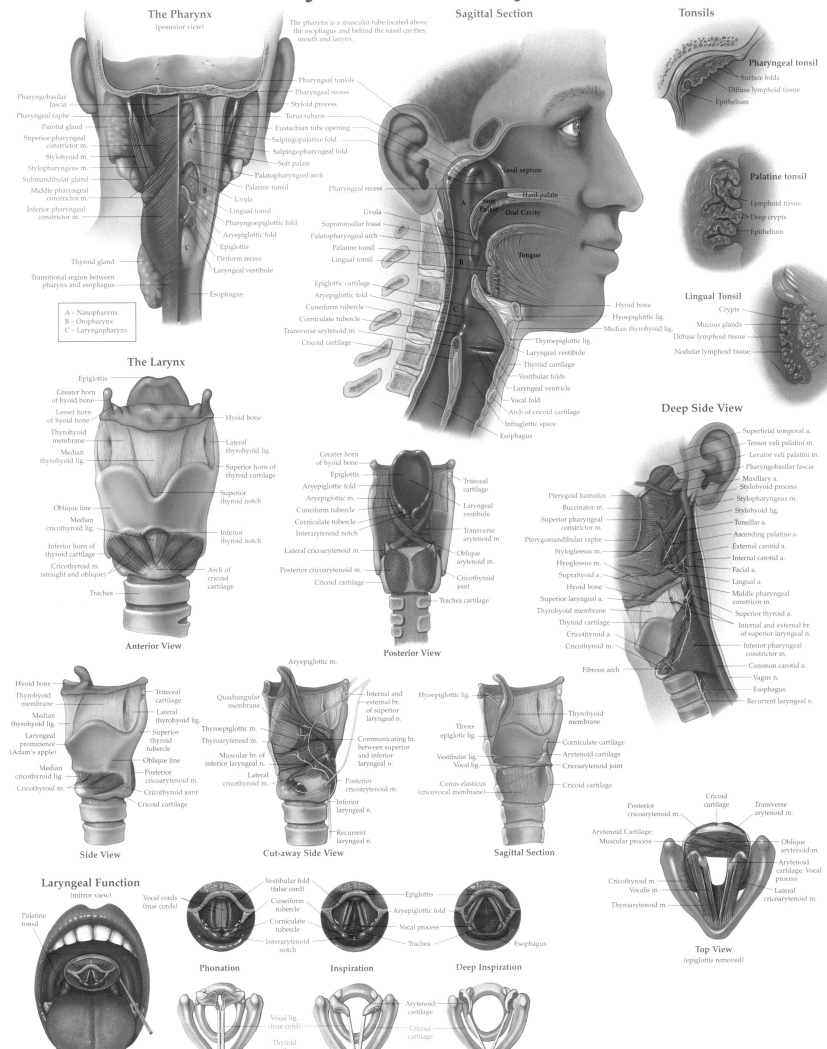

The Pharynx
(posterior view)

The pharynx is a muscular tube located above the esophagus and behind the nasal cavities, mouth and larynx.

Sagittal Section

Tonsils

Pharyngeal tonsils
Pharyngeal recess
Styloid process
Torus tubaris
Eustachian tube opening
Salpingopalatine fold
Salpingopharyngeal fold
Soft palate
Palatopharyngeal arch
Palatine tonsil
Uvula
Lingual tonsil
Pharyngoepiglottic fold
Aryepiglottic fold
Epiglottis
Piriform recess
Laryngeal vestibule
Esophagus

Pharyngobasilar fascia
Pharyngeal raphe
Parotid gland
Superior pharyngeal constrictor m.
Stylohyoid m.
Stylopharyngeus m.
Submandibular gland
Middle pharyngeal constrictor m.
Inferior pharyngeal constrictor m.
Thyroid gland
Transitional region between pharynx and esophagus

A – Nasopharynx
B – Oropharynx
C – Laryngopharynx

Nasal septum
Soft Palate
Hard palate
Oral Cavity
Tongue
Pharyngeal recess
Uvula
Supratonsillar fossa
Palatopharyngeal arch
Palatine tonsil
Lingual tonsil
Epiglottic cartilage
Aryepiglottic fold
Cuneiform tubercle
Corniculate tubercle
Transverse arytenoid m.
Cricoid cartilage

Hyoid bone
Hyoepiglottic lig.
Median thyrohyoid lig.
Thyroepiglottic lig.
Laryngeal vestibule
Thyroid cartilage
Vestibular folds
Laryngeal ventricle
Vocal fold
Arch of cricoid cartilage
Infraglottic space
Esophagus

Pharyngeal tonsil
Surface folds
Diffuse lymphoid tissue
Epithelium

Palatine tonsil
Lymphoid tissue
Deep crypts
Epithelium

Lingual Tonsil
Crypts
Mucous glands
Diffuse lymphoid tissue
Nodular lymphoid tissue

The Larynx

Epiglottis
Greater horn of hyoid bone
Lesser horn of hyoid bone
Thyrohyoid membrane
Median thyrohyoid lig.
Oblique line
Median cricothyroid lig.
Inferior horn of thyroid cartilage
Cricothyroid m. (straight and oblique)
Trachea

Hyoid bone
Lateral thyrohyoid lig.
Superior horn of thyroid cartilage
Superior thyroid notch
Inferior thyroid notch
Arch of cricoid cartilage

Anterior View

Greater horn of hyoid bone
Epiglottis
Aryepiglottic fold
Aryepiglottic m.
Cuneiform tubercle
Corniculate tubercle
Interarytenoid notch
Lateral cricoarytenoid m.
Posterior cricoarytenoid m.
Cricoid cartilage

Triticeal cartilage
Laryngeal vestibule
Transverse arytenoid m.
Oblique arytenoid m.
Cricothyroid joint
Trachea cartilage

Posterior View

Deep Side View

Superficial temporal a.
Tensor veli palatini m.
Levator veli palatini m.
Pharyngobasilar fascia
Maxillary a.
Stylohyoid process
Stylopharyngeus m.
Stylohyoid lig.
Tonsillar a.
Ascending palatine a.
External carotid a.
Internal carotid a.
Facial a.
Lingual a.
Middle pharyngeal constrictor m.
Superior thyroid a.
Internal and external br. of superior laryngeal n.
Inferior pharyngeal constrictor m.
Common carotid a.
Vagus n.
Esophagus
Recurrent laryngeal n.

Pterygoid hamulus
Buccinator m.
Superior pharyngeal constrictor m.
Pterygomandibular raphe
Styloglossus m.
Hyoglossus m.
Suprahyoid a.
Hyoid bone
Superior laryngeal a.
Thyrohyoid membrane
Thyroid cartilage
Cricothyroid a.
Cricothyroid m.
Fibrous arch

Hyoid bone
Thyrohyoid membrane
Median thyrohyoid lig.
Laryngeal prominence (Adam's apple)
Median cricothyroid lig.
Cricothyroid m.

Triticeal cartilage
Lateral thyrohyoid lig.
Superior thyroid tubercle
Oblique line
Posterior cricoarytenoid m.
Cricothyroid joint
Cricoid cartilage

Side View

Aryepiglottic m.
Quadrangular membrane
Thyroepiglottic m.
Thyroarytenoid m.
Muscular br. of inferior laryngeal n.
Lateral cricothyroid m.

Internal and external br. of superior laryngeal n.
Communicating br. between superior and inferior laryngeal n.
Posterior cricoarytenoid m.
Inferior laryngeal n.
Recurrent laryngeal n.

Cut-away Side View

Hyoepiglottic lig.
Thyroepiglotic lig.
Vestibular lig.
Vocal lig.
Conus elasticus (cricovocal membrane)

Thyrohyoid membrane
Corniculate cartilage
Arytenoid cartilage
Cricoarytenoid joint
Cricoid cartilage

Sagittal Section

Posterior cricoarytenoid m.
Arytenoid Cartilage: Muscular process
Cricothyroid m.
Vocalis m.
Thyroarytenoid m.

Cricoid cartilage
Transverse arytenoid m.
Oblique arytenoid m.
Arytenoid cartilage: Vocal process
Lateral cricoarytenoid m.

Top View
(epiglottis removed)

Laryngeal Function
(mirror view)

Palatine tonsil

Vestibular fold (false cord)
Vocal cords (true cords)
Cuneiform tubercle
Corniculate tubercle
Interarytenoid notch

Epiglottis
Aryepiglottic fold
Vocal process
Trachea
Esophagus

Phonation

Inspiration

Deep Inspiration

Vocal lig. (true cord)
Thyroid cartilage
Arytenoid cartilage
Cricoid cartilage

Pregnancy and Birth

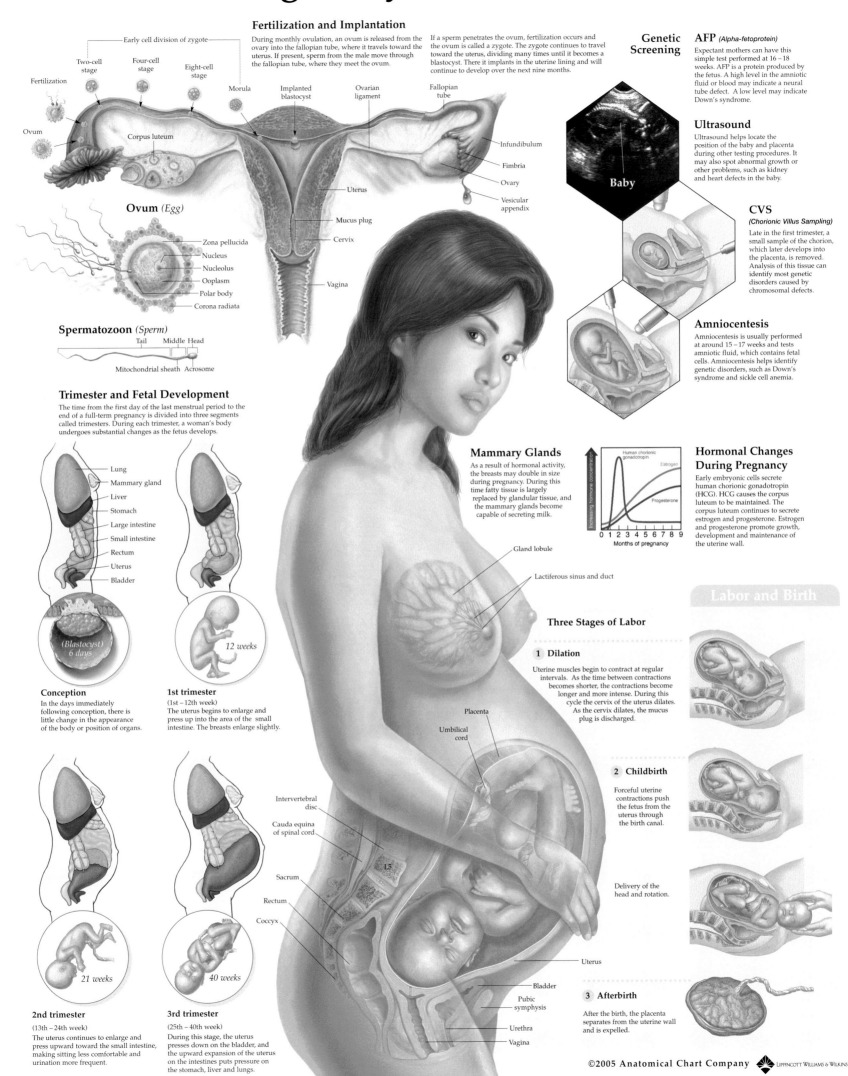

38

Fertilization and Implantation

Early cell division of zygote

Two-cell stage
Four-cell stage
Eight-cell stage

Fertilization

Ovum

Corpus luteum

Morula

Implanted blastocyst

Ovarian ligament

Fallopian tube

Infundibulum

Fimbria

Ovary

Vesicular appendix

Uterus

Mucus plug

Cervix

Vagina

During monthly ovulation, an ovum is released from the ovary into the fallopian tube, where it travels toward the uterus. If present, sperm from the male move through the fallopian tube, where they meet the ovum.

If a sperm penetrates the ovum, fertilization occurs and the ovum is called a zygote. The zygote continues to travel toward the uterus, dividing many times until it becomes a blastocyst. There it implants in the uterine lining and will continue to develop over the next nine months.

Ovum (Egg)

Zona pellucida
Nucleus
Nucleolus
Ooplasm
Polar body
Corona radiata

Spermatozoon (Sperm)

Tail   Middle Head

Mitochondrial sheath   Acrosome

Trimester and Fetal Development

The time from the first day of the last menstrual period to the end of a full-term pregnancy is divided into three segments called trimesters. During each trimester, a woman's body undergoes substantial changes as the fetus develops.

Lung
Mammary gland
Liver
Stomach
Large intestine
Small intestine
Rectum
Uterus
Bladder

(Blastocyst) 6 days

12 weeks

Conception
In the days immediately following conception, there is little change in the appearance of the body or position of organs.

1st trimester
(1st – 12th week)
The uterus begins to enlarge and press up into the area of the small intestine. The breasts enlarge slightly.

21 weeks

40 weeks

2nd trimester
(13th – 24th week)
The uterus continues to enlarge and press upward toward the small intestine, making sitting less comfortable and urination more frequent.

3rd trimester
(25th – 40th week)
During this stage, the uterus presses down on the bladder, and the upward expansion of the uterus on the intestines puts pressure on the stomach, liver and lungs.

Genetic Screening

AFP (Alpha-fetoprotein)
Expectant mothers can have this simple test performed at 16 – 18 weeks. AFP is a protein produced by the fetus. A high level in the amniotic fluid or blood may indicate a neural tube defect. A low level may indicate Down's syndrome.

Baby

Ultrasound
Ultrasound helps locate the position of the baby and placenta during other testing procedures. It may also spot abnormal growth or other problems, such as kidney and heart defects in the baby.

CVS
(Chorionic Villus Sampling)
Late in the first trimester, a small sample of the chorion, which later develops into the placenta, is removed. Analysis of this tissue can identify most genetic disorders caused by chromosomal defects.

Amniocentesis
Amniocentesis is usually performed at around 15 – 17 weeks and tests amniotic fluid, which contains fetal cells. Amniocentesis helps identify genetic disorders, such as Down's syndrome and sickle cell anemia.

Mammary Glands

As a result of hormonal activity, the breasts may double in size during pregnancy. During this time fatty tissue is largely replaced by glandular tissue, and the mammary glands become capable of secreting milk.

Gland lobule

Lactiferous sinus and duct

Hormonal Changes During Pregnancy

Early embryonic cells secrete human chorionic gonadotropin (HCG). HCG causes the corpus luteum to be maintained. The corpus luteum continues to secrete estrogen and progesterone. Estrogen and progesterone promote growth, development and maintenance of the uterine wall.

Human chorionic gonadotropin
Estrogen
Progesterone

0 1 2 3 4 5 6 7 8 9
Months of pregnancy

Three Stages of Labor

1 Dilation
Uterine muscles begin to contract at regular intervals. As the time between contractions becomes shorter, the contractions become longer and more intense. During this cycle the cervix of the uterus dilates. As the cervix dilates, the mucus plug is discharged.

Placenta

Umbilical cord

Labor and Birth

2 Childbirth
Forceful uterine contractions push the fetus from the uterus through the birth canal.

Intervertebral disc

Cauda equina of spinal cord

L5

Delivery of the head and rotation.

Sacrum

Rectum

Coccyx

Uterus

Bladder

Pubic symphysis

3 Afterbirth
After the birth, the placenta separates from the uterine wall and is expelled.

Urethra

Vagina

©2005 Anatomical Chart Company   LIPPINCOTT WILLIAMS & WILKINS

The Prostate

39

Hormonal Influence on the Prostate

The prostate functions continuously, producing fluid which empties into the urethra. Hormones from the **pituitary gland** direct the **adrenal glands** and the **testes** to send chemical signals to the **prostate** to promote fluid production.

- Pituitary
- Adrenal gland
- Kidney
- Ureter
- Urinary bladder
- Prostate
- Testis

What is the Prostate?

The prostate is a gland consisting of fibrous, muscular and glandular tissue surrounding the urethra below the urinary bladder. Its function is to secrete prostatic fluid as a medium for semen, helping it to reach the female reproductive tract. Within the prostate, the urethra is joined by two ejaculatory ducts. During sexual activity, the prostate acts as a valve between the urinary and reproductive tracts. This enables semen to ejaculate without mixing with urine. Prostatic fluid is delivered by the contraction of muscles around gland tissue. Nerve and hormonal influences control the secretory and muscular functions of the prostate.

Posterior View (dissected)

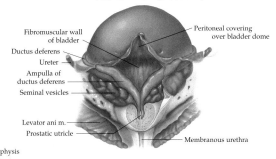

- Fibromuscular wall of bladder
- Ductus deferens
- Ureter
- Ampulla of ductus deferens
- Seminal vesicles
- Levator ani m.
- Prostatic utricle
- Peritoneal covering over bladder dome
- Membranous urethra

Normal Prostate (sagittal section)

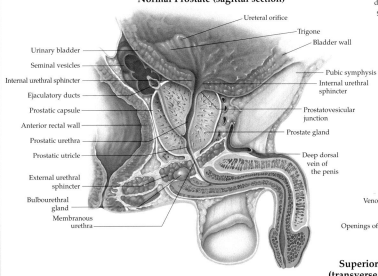

- Ureteral orifice
- Trigone
- Bladder wall
- Urinary bladder
- Seminal vesicles
- Internal urethral sphincter
- Ejaculatory ducts
- Prostatic capsule
- Anterior rectal wall
- Prostatic urethra
- Prostatic utricle
- External urethral sphincter
- Bulbourethral gland
- Membranous urethra
- Pubic symphysis
- Internal urethral sphincter
- Prostatovesicular junction
- Prostate gland
- Deep dorsal vein of the penis

Anterior View with Exposed Prostatic Urethra

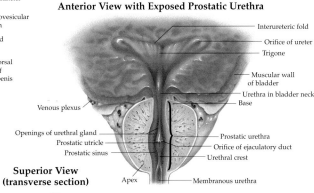

- Interureteric fold
- Orifice of ureter
- Trigone
- Muscular wall of bladder
- Urethra in bladder neck
- Base
- Venous plexus
- Openings of urethral gland
- Prostatic utricle
- Prostatic sinus
- Apex
- Prostatic urethra
- Orifice of ejaculatory duct
- Urethral crest
- Membranous urethra

Superior View (transverse section)

- Prostate glandular tissue lobes
- Prostatic urethra
- Prostatic utricle
- Ejaculatory ducts

Vasculature and Innervation

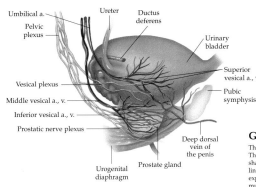

- Umbilical a.
- Pelvic plexus
- Vesical plexus
- Middle vesical a., v.
- Inferior vesical a., v.
- Prostatic nerve plexus
- Ureter
- Ductus deferens
- Urinary bladder
- Superior vesical a., v.
- Pubic symphysis
- Urogenital diaphragm
- Prostate gland
- Deep dorsal vein of the penis

Zones of the Prostate

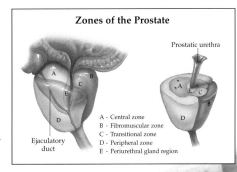

- Prostatic urethra
- Ejaculatory duct
- A - Central zone
- B - Fibromuscular zone
- C - Transitional zone
- D - Peripheral zone
- E - Periurethral gland region

Glands of the Prostate

The prostate is mainly filled with secretory glands. These glands are made of many ducts with grape-shaped saccule ends or "acini". Secretory cells lining the ducts are stimulated by hormones to expel prostatic fluid. During sexual activity muscle contracts and secrete prostatic fluid. The basal cell, also found lining the ducts of the prostate, may be responsible for most types of prostatic hyperplasia as a result of uncontrolled prostatic tissue growth.

Secretory gland with grape-shaped **acinus** end.

- Prostatic duct
- **Secretory cells** are the most numerous in the gland and form the inner lining.
- The **basal cell** is located below the lining surface and may function to rebuild prostatic tissue after infection or other damage.
- Fibromuscular stroma
- Ductal lumen
- Prostatic fluid

Benign Prostatic Hyperplasia (BPH)

Benign Prostatic Hyperplasia (BPH), is the most common type of tumor in mature men. It is a benign growth, which means it may enlarge but will not spread to other locations in the body. The tumor can cause discomfort and may grow to completely close the bladder neck, preventing urination. This condition occurs because the tumor usually grows in the transitional zone and periurethral gland region located at the prostate base near the bladder neck.

Early BPH:

Narrowing of the prostatic urethra causing difficulty in starting, maintaining, and stopping urination.

- Prostatic urethra

Prostatitis

Prostatitis is an uncomfortable condition in which the prostate becomes inflamed and swollen due to an infection. Prostatitis can make urinating painful.

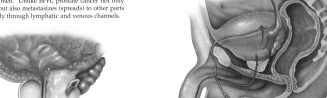

- Prostatis (inflamed prostate tissues)

A **digital rectal exam** is very useful in detecting early signs of prostatic enlargement.

Prostate Cancer

Prostate carcinoma is the most common malignant tumor in men. Unlike BPH, prostate cancer not only enlarges but also metastasizes (spreads) to other parts of the body through lymphatic and venous channels.

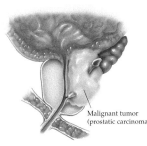

- Malignant tumor (prostatic carcinoma)

Pathways of Prostate Cancer Spread

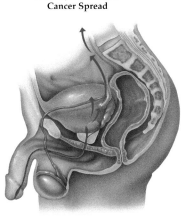

40

Shoulder and Elbow

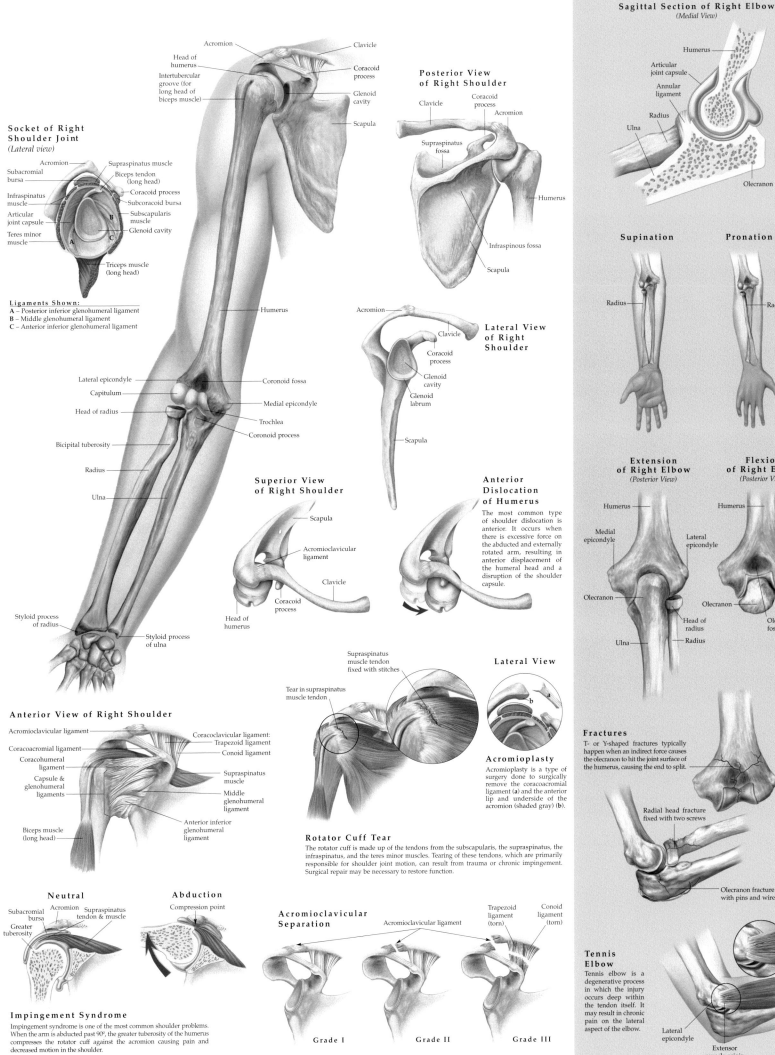

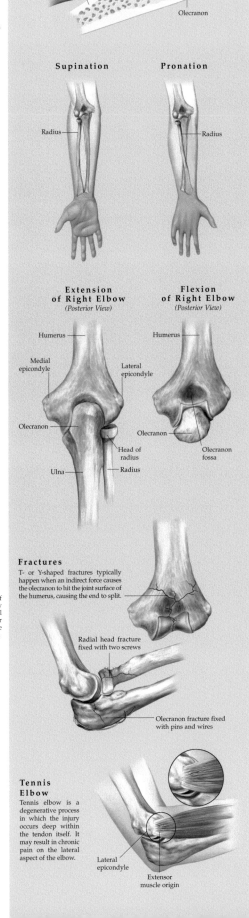

Socket of Right Shoulder Joint
(Lateral view)

Acromion
Subacromial bursa
Infraspinatus muscle
Articular joint capsule
Teres minor muscle
Supraspinatus muscle
Biceps tendon (long head)
Coracoid process
Subcoracoid bursa
Subscapularis muscle
Glenoid cavity
Triceps muscle (long head)

Ligaments Shown:
A – Posterior inferior glenohumeral ligament
B – Middle glenohumeral ligament
C – Anterior inferior glenohumeral ligament

Acromion
Head of humerus
Intertubercular groove (for long head of biceps muscle)
Clavicle
Coracoid process
Glenoid cavity
Scapula
Humerus

Lateral epicondyle
Capitulum
Head of radius
Bicipital tuberosity
Radius
Ulna
Coronoid fossa
Medial epicondyle
Trochlea
Coronoid process

Styloid process of radius
Styloid process of ulna

Posterior View of Right Shoulder

Clavicle
Coracoid process
Acromion
Supraspinatus fossa
Humerus
Infraspinous fossa
Scapula

Lateral View of Right Shoulder

Acromion
Clavicle
Coracoid process
Glenoid cavity
Glenoid labrum
Scapula

Superior View of Right Shoulder

Scapula
Acromioclavicular ligament
Clavicle
Coracoid process
Head of humerus

Anterior Dislocation of Humerus
The most common type of shoulder dislocation is anterior. It occurs when there is excessive force on the abducted and externally rotated arm, resulting in anterior displacement of the humeral head and a disruption of the shoulder capsule.

Anterior View of Right Shoulder

Acromioclavicular ligament
Coracoacromial ligament
Coracohumeral ligament
Capsule & glenohumeral ligaments
Biceps muscle (long head)
Coracoclavicular ligament: Trapezoid ligament
Conoid ligament
Supraspinatus muscle
Middle glenohumeral ligament
Anterior inferior glenohumeral ligament

Supraspinatus muscle tendon fixed with stitches
Tear in supraspinatus muscle tendon

Lateral View

Acromioplasty
Acromioplasty is a type of surgery done to surgically remove the coracoacromial ligament (a) and the anterior lip and underside of the acromion (shaded gray) (b).

Rotator Cuff Tear
The rotator cuff is made up of the tendons from the subscapularis, the supraspinatus, the infraspinatus, and the teres minor muscles. Tearing of these tendons, which are primarily responsible for shoulder joint motion, can result from trauma or chronic impingement. Surgical repair may be necessary to restore function.

Neutral
Subacromial bursa
Acromion
Supraspinatus tendon & muscle
Greater tuberosity

Abduction
Compression point

Acromioclavicular Separation
Acromioclavicular ligament
Trapezoid ligament (torn)
Conoid ligament (torn)
Grade I
Grade II
Grade III

Impingement Syndrome
Impingement syndrome is one of the most common shoulder problems. When the arm is abducted past 90°, the greater tuberosity of the humerus compresses the rotator cuff against the acromion causing pain and decreased motion in the shoulder.

Sagittal Section of Right Elbow
(Medial View)
Humerus
Articular joint capsule
Annular ligament
Radius
Ulna
Olecranon

Supination
Radius

Pronation
Radius

Extension of Right Elbow
(Posterior View)
Humerus
Medial epicondyle
Olecranon
Head of radius
Ulna
Radius

Flexion of Right Elbow
(Posterior View)
Humerus
Lateral epicondyle
Olecranon
Olecranon fossa

Fractures
T- or Y-shaped fractures typically happen when an indirect force causes the olecranon to hit the joint surface of the humerus, causing the end to split.
Radial head fracture fixed with two screws
Olecranon fracture fixed with pins and wires

Tennis Elbow
Tennis elbow is a degenerative process in which the injury occurs deep within the tendon itself. It may result in chronic pain on the lateral aspect of the elbow.
Lateral epicondyle
Extensor muscle origin

 LIPPINCOTT WILLIAMS & WILKINS

41

The Skin and Common Disorders

Normal Anatomy

The skin is the body's largest organ. It covers the entire body and weighs approximately six pounds. The skin includes two primary layers: the outer epidermis and the inner dermis. The epidermis has important protective functions. It protects against injury and excessive water loss. It also prevents disease-causing microorganisms from entering the body.

The thick dermis contains blood vessels, nerve endings, and glands that respond to heat, pressure, and pain. Beneath the dermis, the subcutaneous layer is made up of loose connective tissue and fat (adipose) tissue. This layer acts as a cushion for the skin, helps maintain body heat, and is a store of energy.

Derivatives of Skin

Derivatives of skin include hair, sebaceous glands, sweat glands and nails. These structures all derive from specialized areas of the epidermis that grow down into the dermis.

Hair

Inner root sheath
Huxley's layer
Henle's layer
Medulla
Cortex
Cuticle
Hair shaft
Outer root sheath
Glassy membrane
Connective tissue sheath

Nail

Lateral nail fold
Nail plate
Nail bed
Hyponychium
Lunula
Eponychium
Nail matrix
Nail root

Types of Skin Lesions

Fissure
A painful, cracklike lesion of the skin that extends at least into the dermis.

Ulcer
A craterlike lesion of the skin that usually extends at least into the dermis.

Cyst
A closed sac in or under the skin that contains fluid or semisolid material.

Macule
A small, discolored spot or patch on the skin.

Papule
A solid, raised lesion that is usually less than 1 cm in diameter.

Wheal
A raised reddish area, often itchy, lasting 24 hours or less.

Vesicle
A small fluid filled blister, usually 1 cm or less in diameter.

Pustule
A small, pus filled lesion. If it contains a hair it is called a follicular pustule.

Bulla
A large fluid filled blister, usually 1 cm or more in diameter.

Nodule
A raised lesion detectable by touch, usually 1 cm or more in diameter.

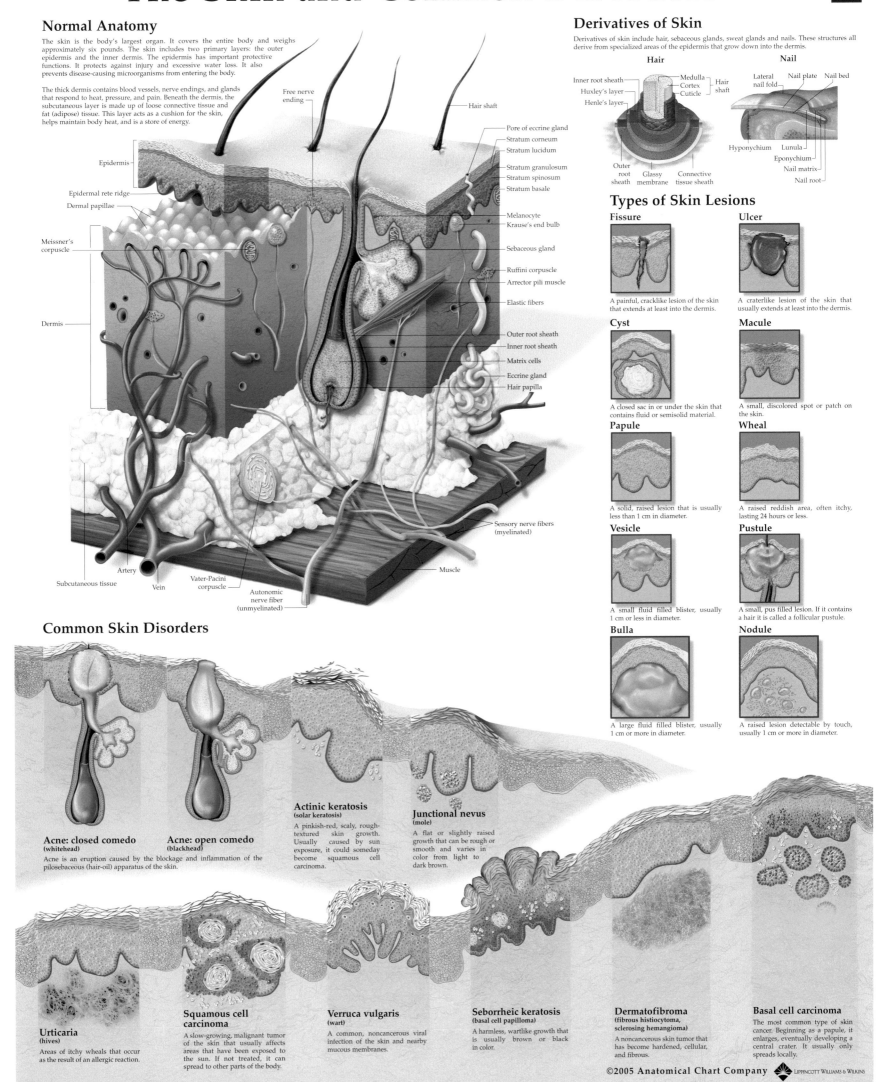

Labels (Normal Anatomy illustration):
Free nerve ending
Hair shaft
Pore of eccrine gland
Stratum corneum
Stratum lucidum
Stratum granulosum
Stratum spinosum
Stratum basale
Melanocyte
Krause's end bulb
Sebaceous gland
Ruffini corpuscle
Arrector pili muscle
Elastic fibers
Outer root sheath
Inner root sheath
Matrix cells
Eccrine gland
Hair papilla
Epidermis
Epidermal rete ridge
Dermal papillae
Meissner's corpuscle
Dermis
Subcutaneous tissue
Artery
Vein
Vater-Pacini corpuscle
Autonomic nerve fiber (unmyelinated)
Sensory nerve fibers (myelinated)
Muscle

Common Skin Disorders

Acne: closed comedo (whitehead)
Acne: open comedo (blackhead)
Acne is an eruption caused by the blockage and inflammation of the pilosebaceous (hair-oil) apparatus of the skin.

Actinic keratosis (solar keratosis)
A pinkish-red, scaly, rough-textured skin growth. Usually caused by sun exposure, it could someday become squamous cell carcinoma.

Junctional nevus (mole)
A flat or slightly raised growth that can be rough or smooth and varies in color from light to dark brown.

Urticaria (hives)
Areas of itchy wheals that occur as the result of an allergic reaction.

Squamous cell carcinoma
A slow-growing, malignant tumor of the skin that usually affects areas that have been exposed to the sun. If not treated, it can spread to other parts of the body.

Verruca vulgaris (wart)
A common, noncancerous viral infection of the skin and nearby mucous membranes.

Seborrheic keratosis (basal cell papilloma)
A harmless, wartlike growth that is usually brown or black in color.

Dermatofibroma (fibrous histiocytoma, sclerosing hemangioma)
A noncancerous skin tumor that has become hardened, cellular, and fibrous.

Basal cell carcinoma
The most common type of skin cancer. Beginning as a papule, it enlarges, eventually developing a central crater. It usually only spreads locally.

©2005 Anatomical Chart Company   LIPPINCOTT WILLIAMS & WILKINS

42

The Spinal Nerves

Portion of Thoracic Spinal Cord with Spinal Nerves
(Diagrammatic)

Anterior gray column
Posterior gray column
Intermediate lateral column
Sympathetic trunk
Paravertebral ganglion
Ventral root (efferent)
Anterior cutaneous branch
Muscular branch
Lateral cutaneous branch
Lateral funiculus
Meningeal ramus
White ramus
Gray ramus
Posterior funiculus
Dorsal root (afferent)
Spinal ganglion
Ventral primary ramus
Dorsal primary ramus
Deep (muscular)
Superficial (cutaneous)

Brain (lateral view, labeled)

Thalamus
I
Olfactory bulb
II
III
IV
V
VI
VIII
VII
IX
X
XI
XII
Greater occipital nerve
C4
Ciliary ganglion
Pterygopalatine ganglion
Trigeminal ganglion

Cranial Nerves

I Olfactory n.	VII Facial n.
II Optic n.	VIII Vestibulocochlear n.
III Oculomotor n.	IX Glossopharyngeal n.
IV Trochlear n.	X Vagus n.
V Trigeminal n.	XI Accessory n.
VI Abducens n.	XII Hypoglossal n.

Spinal Cord Segments

Vertebrae

C1–8   Cervical nerves
T1–12 Thoracic nerves
L1–5   Lumbar nerves
S1–5   Sacral nerves
Co1   Coccygeal nerve

Cervical
C 1 2 3 4 5 6 7 8
T 1 2 3 4 5 6 7 8 9 10 11 12 (Thoracic)
L 1 2 3 4 5 (Lumbar)
S 1 2 3 4 5 (Sacral)
Co 1 (Coccyx)

Lumbar plexus
Sacral plexus

Posterior View (main figure labels)

Minor occipital n.
Great auricular n.
Transverse cervical n.
Supraclavicular n.
Dorsal scapular n.
Suprascapular n.
Long thoracic n. (C5, C6, C7)
Medial pectoral n. (C8, T1)
Medial cutaneous n. of arm and forearm
Musculocutaneous n. (C5, C6, C7)
Axillary n. (C5, C6)
Median n.
Ulnar n.
Radial n. (C5, C6, C7, C8, T1)
Lateral cutaneous n. of forearm
Deep branch of Radial n.
Posterior interosseous n.
Superficial branch of radial n. (C5, C6, C7, C8)
Ulnar n. (C7, C8, T1)
Median n. (C5, C6, C7, C8, T1)
Dorsal digital n.
Median n.

C1 C2 C3 C4 — Cervical plexus
C5 C6 C7 C8 T1 — Brachial plexus

Posterior cord (C5, C6, C7, C8, T1)
Lateral cord (C5, C6, C7)
Medial cord (C8, T1)
Musculocutaneous n.
Axillary n.
Median n. (C5, C6, C7, C8, T1)
T7
Median n.
Ulnar n.
Radial n. (C5, C6, C7, C8, T1)
T12
Iliohypogastric n. (T12, L1)
Ilioinguinal n. (L1)
Genitofemoral n. (L1, L2)
Lateral femoral cutaneous n. (L2, L3)
Femoral n. (L2, L3, L4)
Obturator n. (L2, L3, L4)
Superior gluteal n. (L4, L5, S1)
Inferior gluteal n. (L5, S1, S2)
Sciatic n. (L4, L5, S1, S2, S3)
Common peroneal n. (posterior division of ventral rami) (L4, L5, S1, S2)
Tibial n. (anterior division of ventral rami) (L4, L5, S1, S2, S3)
Median n.
Ulnar n.
Pudendal n. (S2, S3, S4)

L1 L2 L3 L4 L5 S1 S2 S3 S4 S5 Co1

Posterior femoral cutaneous n. (S1, S2, S3)
Tibial n. (L4, L5, S1, S2, S3)
Common peroneal n. (L4, L5, S1, S2)
Lateral sural cutaneous n.
Medial sural cutaneous n.
Saphenous n.
Tibial n.

Cutaneous Distribution of the Spinal Nerves (Anterior View)

Ophthalmic n.
Maxillary n.
Mandibular n.
Greater occipital n.
Lesser occipital n.
Great auricular n.
Transverse cervical n.
Intercostals:
Anterior cutaneous n.
Lateral cutaneous
Supraclavicular n.
Axillary n.
Medial brachial cutaneous n. and intercostobrachial n.
Radial n.
Antebrachial cutaneous nerves:
Posterior
Lateral
Ulnar n.
Radial n.
Median n.
Iliohypogastric n.
Ilioinguinal n.
Genitofemoral n.
Lateral femoral cutaneous n.
Anterior femoral cutaneous n.
Obturator n.
Saphenous n.
Lateral sural cutaneous n.
Superficial peroneal n.
Sural n.
Deep peroneal n.

Cutaneous Distribution of the Spinal Nerves (Posterior View)

Greater occipital n.
Great auricular n.
Lesser occipital n.
Supraclavicular n.
Dorsal rami of thoracic nn.
Axillary n.
Medial brachial cutaneous n. and intercostobrachial n.
Radial n.
Antebrachial cutaneous nerves:
Lateral
Posterior
Medial
Ulnar n.
Radial n.
Median n.
Iliohypogastric n.
Superior cluneal n.
Inferior cluneal n.
Lateral femoral cutaneous n.
Posterior femoral cutaneous n.
Obturator n.
Lateral sural cutaneous n.
Medial sural cutaneous n.
Saphenous n.
Plantar branches of tibial n.

Dermal Segmentation (Dermatomes)

C1 C2 C3 C4 C5 C6 C7 C8
T1 T2 T3 T4 T5 T6 T7 T8 T9 T10 T11 T12
L1 L2 L3 L4 L5
S1 S2 S3

Anatomy of the Teeth

43

Primary Teeth

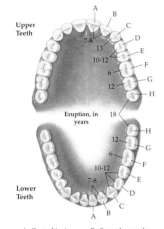

Upper Teeth

A
B
C
F
G
6
7-8
16
12
24

Eruption, in months

Lower Teeth

24
12
16
7-8
6
G
F
C
A
B

Permanent Teeth

Upper Teeth

A
B
C
D
E
F
G
H
7-8
13
10-12
6
12

Eruption, in years   18

Lower Teeth

H
12
6
10-12
7-8
G
F
E
D
C
A
B

A Central incisor
B Lateral incisor
C Canine
D First premolar
E Second premolar
F First molar
G Second molar
H Third molar

Function of the Teeth

Incisor: Acts like scissors; grasps and cuts food.

Bicuspid: Has two pointed projections; tears, shreds, crushes food.

Cuspid: Has a single, very long, sharp cusp; tears and shreds food.

Molar: Strongest, most useful type of tooth; grinds food into tiny pieces.

1 Enamel
2 Dentin, with dentinal tubules
3 Pulp chamber containing vessels and nerves
4 Gingival (gum) epithelium
5 Lamina propria of gingiva (gum)
6 Bone
7 Periodontium
8 Periodontal membranes
9 Root canal
10 Interradicular septum
11 Apical foramina
12 Odontoblast layer
13 Cementum
14 Gingival sulcus

Childhood Dentition

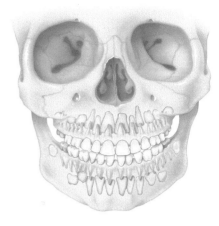

Beneath the erupted primary (baby or milk) teeth lie the permanent teeth (shown in blue). The twenty primary teeth are replaced as the child grows. Eruption and shedding dates are shown in the drawings on the far left.

Oral Cavity

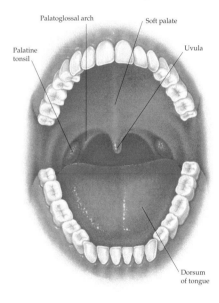

Palatoglossal arch
Soft palate
Palatine tonsil
Uvula
Dorsum of tongue

Tooth Decay

1 Decay of enamel
2 Decay invades dentin
3 Inflammation of pulp
4 Death of pulp
5 Abscess formation

Innervation and Blood Supply

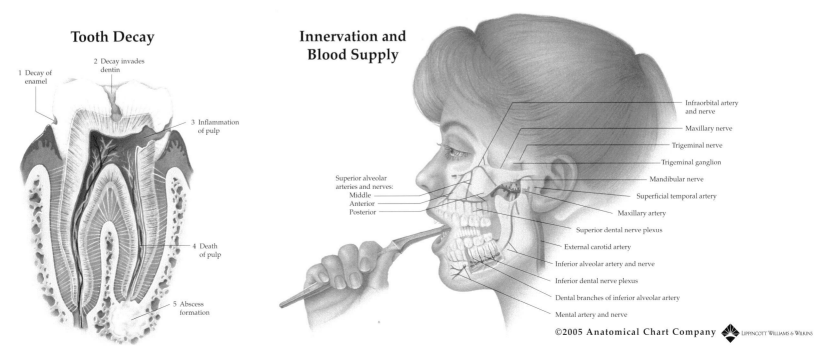

Infraorbital artery and nerve
Maxillary nerve
Trigeminal nerve
Trigeminal ganglion
Mandibular nerve
Superficial temporal artery
Maxillary artery
Superior dental nerve plexus
External carotid artery
Inferior alveolar artery and nerve
Inferior dental nerve plexus
Dental branches of inferior alveolar artery
Mental artery and nerve

Superior alveolar arteries and nerves:
Middle
Anterior
Posterior

©2005 Anatomical Chart Company   LIPPINCOTT WILLIAMS & WILKINS

The Vertebral Column

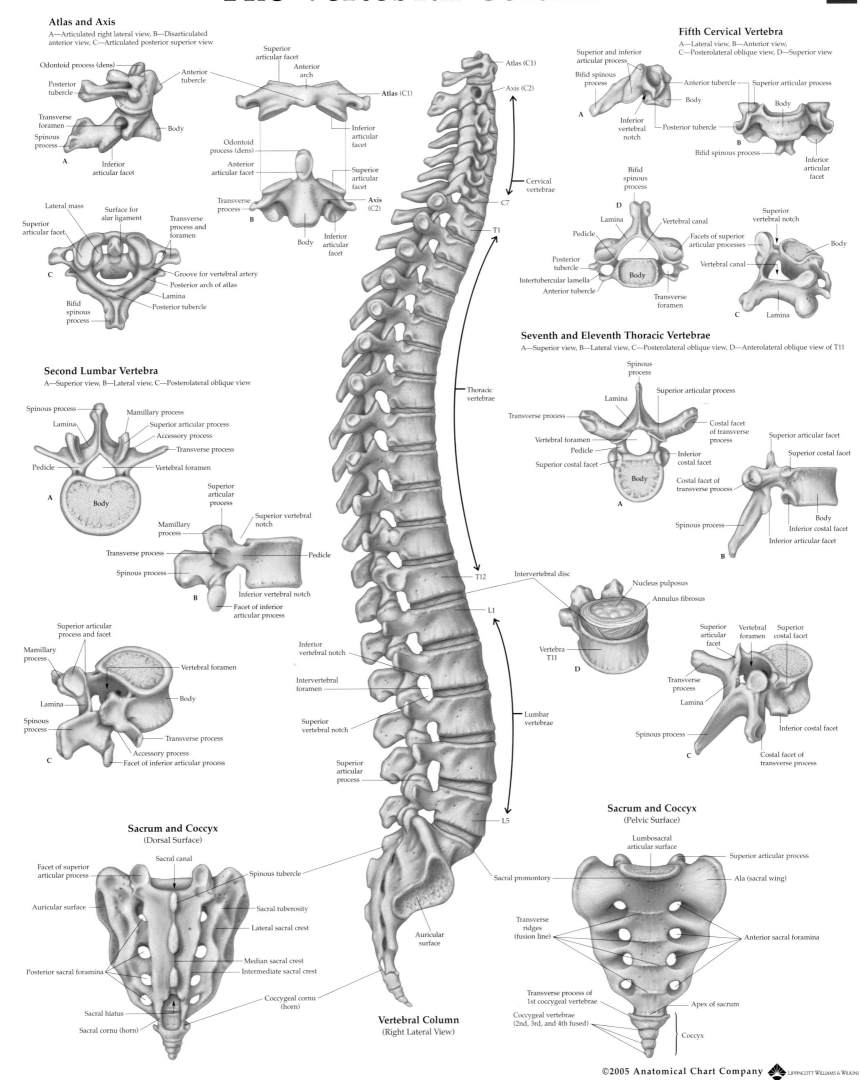